HERBAL ESSENCE

HERBAL ESSENCE

AUTHOR'S
CHANNEL

Dr. Nikhil Govind

ISBN: 978-93-92546-35-8

Published by

AUTHOR'S CHANNEL

Author's Channel

#108, 1st floor, 3rd cross, 3rd stage, 8th Main, Pillanna Garden, Bangalore 560045

Acknowledgement

With a humble heart, I acknowledge the boundless grace of God, whose blessings illuminate my path.

I express my profound gratitude to my parents, **Smt. M. Varalakshmi** and **Sri G. M. Govindappa**, my dearest wife **Rohini Das**, and my family.

I also extend my sincere gratitude to my **Chairman, Dr. Shashi Kumar V. M., Principal Dr. Sumana Bhatt, the lecturers of TMCNYS, and all the teachers who taught me.**

I sincerely express my gratitude to **M. V. Muniraju Sir, Chairman of MVM Educational Institutions, and Dr. Vinutha Rao, Principal of MVMCNYS**, for their continuous support and encouragement.

I am grateful to all my colleagues and students from **MVMCNYS Institute**.

I would like to acknowledge and thank **Ms. Harshitha M., Dr. Sowjanya D., Dr. Ansa Anet Philip, Dr. Chandini, Dr. Sandhya Dattatri, and Ms. K. R. Rohini Das**, the Chief Editor, along with my colleagues in the **Department of BNYS at MVM Educational Institutions**, for their support and assistance.

Dr. Nikhil Govind
Author

Preface

Nature has always been the greatest healer known to humankind. Long before the development of modern medicine, people relied on plants, herbs, and their natural extracts to maintain health and restore balance to the body and mind. Among these natural healing methods, **aromatherapy** stands as one of the most gentle, effective, and holistic systems of healing. The therapeutic use of aromatic plant extracts has been practiced for thousands of years in various cultures including ancient Egypt, India, China, and Greece.

The book **"Herbal Essence"** has been written with the intention of introducing readers to the fascinating world of aromatherapy and the healing power of essential oils derived from herbs and plants. Aromatherapy is not merely about pleasant fragrances; it is a science and an art that works through the sense of smell and skin absorption to influence physical health, emotional balance, and mental well-being. The essential oils used in aromatherapy contain the life force of plants, carrying powerful therapeutic properties that can help the body heal naturally.

In recent years, the interest in natural therapies has grown rapidly. People are increasingly seeking alternatives that are safe, natural, and supportive of the body's own healing mechanisms. Aromatherapy plays an important role in this movement toward holistic health. When used correctly, essential oils can help relieve stress, improve sleep, reduce pain, enhance immunity, and promote relaxation and rejuvenation.

This book aims to present aromatherapy in a clear, practical, and educational manner. It covers the history, principles, extraction methods, properties of essential oils, therapeutic applications, safety guidelines, and practical uses in daily life. Special attention has been given to commonly used essential oils and their benefits in promoting physical and psychological wellness. The information provided in this book is intended to serve students, practitioners of naturopathy, wellness enthusiasts, and anyone interested in understanding natural healing through plant essences.

"Herbal Essence" is not only a guide to aromatherapy but also a tribute to the healing gifts of nature. By understanding and respecting these natural remedies, we can reconnect with traditional wisdom while applying it in modern lifestyles. My hope is that this book will inspire readers to appreciate the therapeutic value of herbs and essential oils and to use them responsibly for health, harmony, and holistic living.

I sincerely hope that **"Herbal Essence"** will serve as a useful resource for learners and practitioners alike. If this work helps even a small number of people understand and benefit from the healing power of aromatherapy, the purpose of writing this book will be fulfilled.

Dr. Nikhil Govind
Author

Dedication

This book *"Herbal Essence"* is humbly dedicated to the **Almighty God**, whose divine blessings, wisdom, and guidance have been the constant light in my journey. It is through His grace that I have been given the strength, inspiration, and opportunity to complete this work.

I lovingly dedicate this book to **my beloved parents**, whose unconditional love, sacrifices, encouragement, and values have shaped my life and supported me in every step of my journey. Their faith in me has always been my greatest motivation.

I extend my heartfelt gratitude and dedicate this work to **my respected teachers and mentors**, who have shared their knowledge, wisdom, and guidance. Their teachings have not only enriched my academic path but have also inspired me to pursue learning and service in the field of natural healing.

I also dedicate this book to **my dear friends**, whose constant support, encouragement, and companionship have made this journey meaningful and memorable.

May this work stand as a small token of my gratitude to all those who have guided, supported, and inspired me throughout my life.

Dr. Nikhil Govind
Author

Table of Contents

Chapter 1
Introduction and History

Aromatherapy is a natural healing therapy that uses essential oils extracted from plants to promote physical, mental, and emotional well-being. These aromatic oils are obtained from different parts of plants such as flowers, leaves, bark, roots, seeds, and fruits.

The term *Aromatherapy* was first coined by the French chemist René-Maurice Gattefossé in the early 20th century after he discovered the healing properties of lavender oil on burns.

Definitions:

1. Aromatherapy is a holistic treatment, utilising esselntial oil extracted from aromatic plant to create balance and harmony of the body, mind and spirit
2. Aromatherapy is a skilled use of essential oil which have been extracted from flowers, spices, fruits, wood & leaves for their aesthetic, psychological & medicinal applications
3. It uses aroma for healing and works on multiple levels. It can treat emotional and physical problems, boost athletic performance, and enhance your love life.
4. The inhaled aroma from the essential oil is widely believed to stimulate brain function. Essential oil can also be absorbed from skin where they travel through the blood stream and can promote whole body healing.
5. *A holistic healing treatment that uses natural plant extracts, often called essential oil therapy. It's considered both an art and a science*

6. According to Oxford Dictionary, *The use of aromatic plant extracts and essential oils for healing and cosmetic purposes.*

Origin of Aromatherapy

Ancient Egypt

The use of essential oils in Ancient Egypt dates back over 5,000 years, reflecting their deep reverence for nature's healing gifts. Egyptians incorporated these aromatic oils into nearly every facet of life—from sacred religious ceremonies and elaborate beauty rituals to practical medicinal treatments. They believed that essential oils possessed potent therapeutic properties, capable of alleviating various ailments and promoting overall well-being. Among the most valued oils were Rose, Frankincense, and Calamus, each prized for its unique fragrance and healing benefits. This holistic approach to health and spirituality underscores the sophistication of Egyptian culture and its enduring legacy in Natural medicine.

China and India

The use of aromatherapy in China and India can be traced back over 3,000 years, reflecting the deep-rooted traditions of natural healing in both cultures. In ancient China, Essential oils were primarily employed for medicinal purposes, with aromatic extracts like Cinnamon and Huang ti valued for their therapeutic effects. Meanwhile, in India, aromatherapy formed an integral part of Ayurveda—the traditional system of medicine focused on balancing the body's energies, or doshas. Oils derived from herbs such as Sandalwood, Ginger, and Jasmine were commonly used in massages, baths, and inhalations to support both physical and emotional well-being. These practices highlight the sophisticated understanding of holistic health in early Eastern civilizations.

The Influence of Traditional Chinese Medicine on Aromatherapy Practices

Traditional Chinese Medicine (TCM) has played a pivotal role in shaping the development and practices of aromatherapy, with its roots extending back thousands of years. Central to TCM is the belief that aromatic herbs and plants possess powerful therapeutic properties capable of influencing the body's vital energy, or **Qi**. Scents were carefully selected to harmonize internal imbalances, calm the spirit, and support physical health. This ancient wisdom not only guided the use of essential oils in traditional healing rituals but also laid the groundwork for their integration into contemporary holistic therapies. Today, many aromatherapy practices continue to draw from TCM principles, emphasizing the energetic and emotional dimensions of scent in promoting overall well-being.

Aromatic Herbs in Traditional Chinese Medicine

In Traditional Chinese Medicine (TCM), aromatic herbs such as Ginger, Cinnamon, and Peppermint have long been valued for their potent medicinal properties. These herbs are commonly brewed into herbal teas or incorporated into remedies aimed at addressing a wide range of health concerns, from digestive issues to respiratory ailments. Beyond their physiological benefits, the distinctive fragrances of these botanicals are believed to influence the body's meridians and internal organs, promoting energetic balance and harmony. Essential oils extracted from these herbs are frequently used in complementary therapies such as Acupuncture and Massage, where their aromatic and therapeutic qualities enhance the overall healing experience. This integrative approach reflects TCM's holistic philosophy, where scent and touch work together to restore wellness.

Aromatherapy Techniques in Traditional Chinese Medicine

In Traditional Chinese Medicine (TCM), aromatherapy techniques are seamlessly integrated into healing modalities to amplify therapeutic outcomes. One such practice is **Moxibustion**, which involves burning dried mugwort leaves to produce aromatic smoke believed to stimulate the flow of **Qi** and support the body's natural healing processes. Additionally, essential oils are often applied to specific **acupressure points**, where their unique properties help address targeted ailments and restore energetic balance. By combining the sensory power of scent with traditional techniques like acupuncture and massage, TCM practitioners enhance the depth and efficacy of treatment. This fusion of aromatherapy with ancient Chinese healing principles reflects a holistic approach aimed at promoting comprehensive wellness and harmony.

Modern Integration of TCM Principles in Aromatherapy

As interest in holistic healing continues to grow, modern practitioners of aromatherapy are blending traditional Chinese medicine principles with contemporary aromatherapy practices. This fusion allows for a more comprehensive approach to health and well-being by addressing both physical symptoms and emotional well-being through the use of essential oils and aromatic blends.

By understanding the historical roots of traditional Chinese medicine within aromatherapy, practitioners can offer a more holistic approach to healing that honors ancient wisdom while embracing modern scientific advancements.

Greece and Rome

The Greeks and Romans also used essential oils for medicinal purposes. Greek mythology mentions the use of essential oils. Hippocrates, the father of modern medicine, used aromatherapy as part of his treatments. The Romans used essential oils in their public baths and believed that they had medicinal properties. The Roman physician, Dioscorides, wrote about the use of essential oils in his book "De Materia Medica."

Aromatherapy has a rich history that dates back thousands of years. From Ancient Egypt to Greece and Rome, essential oils have been used for their therapeutic properties. The use of aromatherapy continues to this day, and its popularity is on the rise.

Aromatherapy in the Middle Ages

During the Middle Ages, aromatherapy continued to be a popular practice. During this time, Avicenna, a physician and philosopher, introduced the process of distillation, which is still used today to extract essential oils from herbs, plants, and fruits. He also wrote extensive instructions on how to use plants and essential oils, including massage to support health.

Islamic Influence

Islamic scholars played a significant role in the development of aromatherapy during the Middle Ages. They translated the works of Greek and Roman physicians and combined them with their own knowledge of medicine, botany, and alchemy. The Islamic Golden Age was a period of great intellectual and cultural growth, and it was during this time that many of the essential oils we use today were first discovered and extracted.

European Practices

In Europe, aromatherapy was primarily used by the clergy and the wealthy. The use of aromatic herbs and oils was seen as a way to purify the body and the soul. The Catholic Church also used aromatherapy in their religious rituals, such as anointing oils for the sick. Latin was the language of the Church, and many of the essential oils used in aromatherapy today still have Latin names.

During the Black Death, which ravaged Europe in the 14th century, aromatherapy was used as a form of antiseptic protection. The Knights of Crusades brought aromatic essences to Europe, and herbs like cinnamon and cloves were placed in a mask over doctors faces in an attempt to filter the air.

In conclusion, aromatherapy was an important part of medicine and culture during the Middle Ages. Islamic scholars played a significant role in its development, and it was used by both the clergy and the wealthy in Europe. Today, we still use many of the essential oils that were first discovered and extracted during this time.

Modern Aromatherapy

Modern aromatherapy has its roots in the work of French chemist René-Maurice Gattefossé, who is credited with coining the term “aromatherapy” in the early 20th century. Gattefossé discovered the healing properties of lavender oil when he applied it to a burn on his hand and found that it healed quickly and without scarring. He went on to study the properties of other essential oils and their effects on the body and mind.

French Influence

Another influential personality in the development of modern aromatherapy is Jean Valnet, a French physician who used essential oils in the treatment of wounded soldiers during World War II. Valnet's work helped to establish the scientific basis for aromatherapy and its use in modern medicine. Today, France remains a major center for the production of essential oils, particularly in the region of Grasse.

Global Expansion

Aromatherapy has since expanded globally, with practitioners and researchers around the world exploring the potential benefits of essential oils. In England, modern aromatherapy was developed by Pierre Franchomme, who studied under Valnet and established the first aromatherapy clinic in the country. Today, aromatherapy is used in a variety of settings, from spas and wellness centres to hospitals and the pharmaceutical industry.

While essential oils are not a substitute for modern medicine, they are increasingly recognized for their potential therapeutic benefits. Research has shown that certain essential oils can help to reduce stress and anxiety, improve sleep quality, and alleviate pain and inflammation. As interest in natural and complementary therapies continues to grow, aromatherapy is likely to play an increasingly important role in promoting health and well-being.

Chapter 2
Extraction methods of Natural essential oils

Essential oils are aromatic volatile liquids distilled from shrubs, flowers, trees, bushes & seeds which contain highly oxygenated molecules.

Essential oils are incorporated into a broad spectrum of consumer products, including detergents, soaps, personal care items, cosmetics, pharmaceuticals, perfumes, confectionery, soft drinks, alcoholic beverages, and insecticides.

Mechanism of Distillation

Hydrodistillation of plant material involves the following main physicochemical processes:

i) *Hydrodiffusion*: Diffusion of essential oils and hot water through plant membranes is known as hydrodiffusion.

ii) *Hydrolysis*: Hydrolysis in the present context is defined as a chemical reaction between water and certain constituents of essential oils.

iii) *Decomposition by heat*: Almost all constituents of essential oils are unstable at high temperature. To obtain the best quality oil, distillation must be done at low temperatures. The temperature in steam distillation is determined entirely by the operating pressure, whereas in water distillation and in water and steam distillation, the operating pressure is usually atmospheric. The rate of diffusion usually increases with temperatures as does the solubility of essential oils in water.

Methods of Producing Essential Oils

There are three types of hydrodistillation

- Water distillation
- Water and steam distillation
- Direct steam distillation

Although the theoretical framework governing two-phase distillation remains consistent across all three methods, the primary distinctions arise from how the plant material is managed during the process.

Water distillation

The material is completely immersed in water which is boiled by applying heat by direct fire, steam jacket, closed steam jacket/open steam coil.

Main characteristics of this method is direct contact between boiling water & plant material.

Requires large amount of steam & is uneconomical.

Still Operation Guidelines

- *Insulation*: Essential to prevent heat loss and water condensation.
- *Agitation*: Crucial during boiling to avoid settling and thermal degradation of dense plant material.
- *Powdering*: Especially for mucilage-rich materials like cinnamon bark, to ensure even dispersion.

During water distillation, all parts of the plant charge must be kept in motion by boiling water; this is possible when the distillation material is charged loosely and remains loose in the boiling water.

For this reason only, water distillation possesses one distinct advantage, i.e. that it permits processing of finely powdered material or plant parts that, by contact with live steam, would otherwise form lumps through which the steam cannot penetrate. Other practical advantages of water distillation is that the stills are inexpensive, easy to construct and suitable for field operation. These are still widely used with portable equipment in many countries.

Disadvantages of Water Distillation

- Oil components like esters are sensitive to hydrolysis while others like acyclic monoterpene hydrocarbons and aldehydes are susceptible to polymerization (since the pH of water is often reduced during distillation, hydrolytic reactions are facilitated).

- Oxygenated components such as phenols have a tendency to dissolve in the still water, so their complete removal by distillation is not possible.

- As water distillation tends to be a small operation (operated by one or two persons), it takes a long time to accumulate much oil, so good quality oil is often mixed with bad quality oil.

- The distillation process is treated as an art by local distillers, who rarely try to optimize both oil yield or quality.

- Water distillation is a slower process than either water and steam distillation or direct steam distillation.

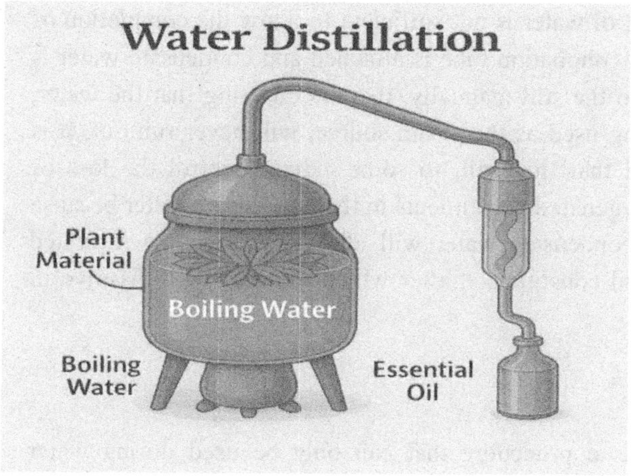

Water and Steam distillation

In water and steam distillation, the steam can be generated either in a satellite boiler or within the still, although separated from the plant material. Like water distillation, water and steam distillation is widely used in rural areas. Moreover, it does not require a great deal more capital expenditure than water distillation. Also, the equipment used is generally similar to that used in water distillation, but the plant material is supported above the boiling water on a perforated grid.

In fact, it is common that persons performing water distillation eventually progress to water and steam distillation. It follows that once rural distillers have produced a few batches of oil by water distillation, they realize that the quality of oil is not very good because of its still notes (subdued aroma). As a result, some modifications are made. Using the same still, a perforated grid or plate is fashioned so that the plant material is raised above the water. This reduces the capacity of the still but affords a better quality of oil.

If the amount of water is not sufficient to allow the completion of distillation, a cohobation tube is attached and condensate water is added back to the still manually, thereby ensuring that the water, which is being used as the steam source, will never run out. It is also believed that this will, to some extent, control the loss of dissolved oxygenated constituents in the condensate water because the re-used condensate water will allow it to become saturated with dissolved constituents, after which more oil will dissolve in it.

Cohobation

Cohobation is a procedure that can only be used during water distillation or water and steam distillation. It uses the practice of returning the distillate water to the still after the oil has been separated from it so that it can be re-boiled. The principle behind it is to minimize the losses of oxygenated components, particularly phenols which dissolve to some extent in the distillate water. For most oils, this level of oil loss through solution in water is less than 0.2%, whereas for phenol-rich oils the amount of oil dissolved in the distillate water is 0.2%-0.7%. As this material is being constantly re-vaporized, condensed and re-vaporized again, any dissolved oxygenated constituents will promote hydrolysis and degradation of themselves or other oil constituents. Similarly, if an oxygenated component is constantly brought in contact with a direct heat source or side of a still, which is considerably hotter than 100° C, then the chances of degradation are enhanced.

As a result, the practice of cohobation is not recommended unless the temperature to which oxygenated constituents in the distillate are exposed is no higher than 100° C.

Advantages of Water and Steam Distillation over Water Distillation

- Higher oil yield.

- Components of the volatile oil are less susceptible to hydrolysis and polymerization (the control of wetness on the bottom of the still affects hydrolysis, whereas the thermal conductivity of the still walls affects polymerization).

- If refluxing is controlled, then the loss of polar compounds are minimized.

- Oil quality produced by steam and water distillation is more reproducible.

- Steam and water distillation is faster than water distillation, so it is more energy efficient. Many oils are currently produced by steam and water distillation, for example lemongrass is produced in Bhutan with a rural steam and water distillation system.

Disadvantages of Water and Steam Distillation

- Due to the low pressure of rising steam, oils of high-boiling range require a greater quantity of steam for vaporization - hence longer hours of distillation.

- The plant material becomes wet, which slows down distillation as the steam has to vaporize the water to allow it to condense further up the still.

- To avoid that the lower plant material resting on the grid becomes waterlogged, a baffle is used to prevent the water from boiling too vigorously and coming in direct contact with the plant material.

Direct Steam Distillation

- Definition: A method where steam is generated externally in a satellite boiler and directed into the still containing plant material.

- Setup: Plant material rests on a perforated grid above the steam inlet, allowing steam to pass through and extract volatile oils

- A feature of direct steam distillation is that steam is generated externally in a satellite boiler, allowing precise control over steam flow and ensuring the plant material is heated to no more than 100°C. This prevents thermal degradation of sensitive compounds, making it ideal for large-scale essential oil production in the flavor and fragrance industry.

Industrial Relevance

- Widely used in the flavor and fragrance industry.

- Preferred for large-scale essential oil production due to its efficiency and quality preservation.

Examples of Low-Cost Oils Often Distilled

★ Rosemary
★ Chinese cedarwood
★ Lemongrass
★ Litsea cubeba
★ Spike lavender
★ Eucalyptus
★ Citronella
★ Cornmint

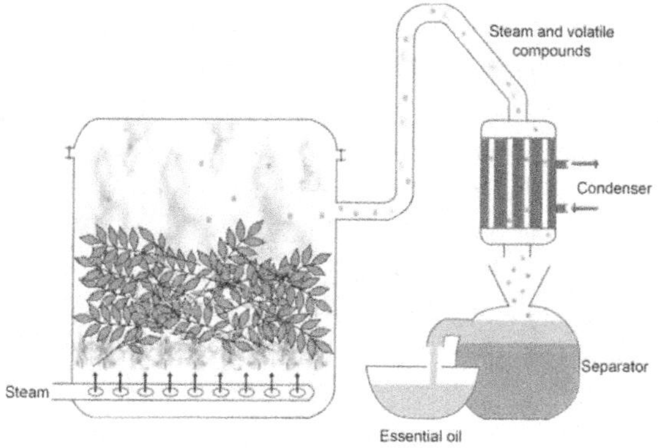

Advantages of Direct Steam Distillation

- The amount of steam can be readily controlled.
- No thermal decomposition of oil constituents.
- Most widely accepted process for large-scale oil production, superior to the other two processes.

Disadvantage of Direct Steam Distillation

- Much higher capital expenditure needed to establish this activity than for the other two processes.

Essential Oil Extraction by Expression

Expression or cold pressing, as it is also known, is only used in the production of citrus oils. The term expression refers to any physical process in which the essential oil glands in the peel are crushed or broken to release the oil. One method that was practiced many years ago, particularly in Sicily (spugna method), commenced with halving the citrus fruit followed by pulp removal with the aid of sharpened spoon-knife (known as a rastrello). The oil was removed from the peel either by pressing the peel against a hard object of baked clay (concolina) which was placed under a large natural sponge or by bending the peel into the sponge. The oil emulsion absorbed by the sponge was removed by squeezing it into the concolina or some other container. It is reported that oil produced this way contains more of the fruit odor character than oil produced by any other method.

A second method known as equaling (or the scodella method), uses a shallow bowl of copper (or sometimes brass) with a hollow central tube; the equaling tool is similar in shape to a shallow funnel. The bowl is equipped with brass points with blunt ends across which the whole citrus fruit is rolled by hand with some pressure until all of the oil glands have burst. The oil and aqueous cell contents are allowed to dribble down the hollow tube into a container from which the oil is separated by decantation.

Obviously, hand pressing is impractical because it is an extremely slow process, e.g. on average only 2-4 lbs oil per day can be produced by a single person using one of these hand methods. As a result, over the years a number of machines have been designed to either crush the peel of a citrus fruit or crush the whole fruit and then separate the oil from the juice.

Pelatrice Process

In the pelatrice process, citrus fruits are fed from a hopper into the abrasive shell of the machine. The fruits are rotated against the abrasive shell by a slow-moving Archimedian screw whose surface rasps the fruit surfaces causing some of the essential oil cavities on the peel to burst and release their oil-water emulsion. This screw further transports the fruit into a hopper in which rollers covered with abrasive spikes burst the remaining oil cavities. The oil and water emulsion is washed away from the fruit by a fine spray of water. The emulsion next passes through a separator where any solids are removed, after which it passes through two centrifugal separators working in series to yield the pure oil. Most bergamot oil and some lemon oil are produced this way in Italy.

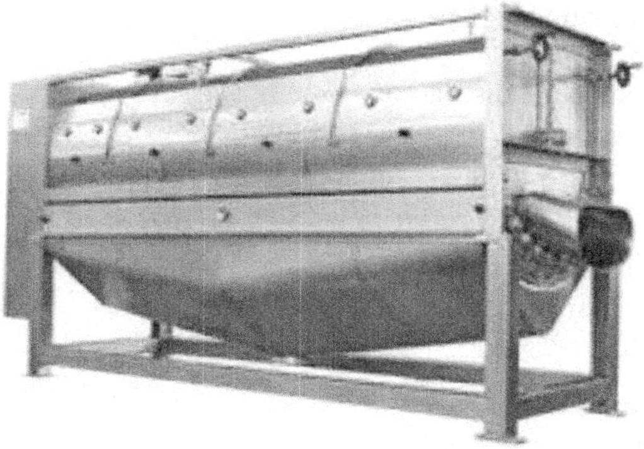

Modern (Non-traditional) Methods of Extraction of Essential Oils

Traditional methods of extraction of essential oils have been discussed and these are the methods most widely used on a commercial scale. However, with technological advancement, new techniques have been developed which may not necessarily be widely used for commercial production of essential oils but are considered valuable in certain situations, such as the production of costly essential oils in a natural state without any alteration of their thermosensitive components or the extraction of essential oils for micro-analysis. These techniques are as follows:

- Headspace trapping techniques

  - Static headspace technique
  - Vacuum headspace technique
  - Dynamic headspace technique
- Solid phase micro-extraction (SPME)
- Supercritical fluid extraction (SFE)
- Phytosol (phytol) extraction
- Protoplast technique
- Simultaneous distillation extraction (SDE)
- Microwave distillation
- Controlled instantaneous decomposition (CID)
- Thermomicrodistillation
- Microdistillation
- Molecular spinning band distillation
- Membrane extraction

Chapter 3
Storage of Aroma Oil

Use Dark Glass Bottles

- Amber or cobalt blue glass protects oils from UV light, which can degrade their quality.
- Avoid plastic containers—essential oils can dissolve plastic and become contaminated.

Keep in a Cool, Stable Temperature

- Ideal range: 10–25°C (50–77°F)
- Avoid heat sources like sunlight, stoves, or radiators.
- Refrigeration is okay for some oils (e.g., citrus oils), but let them return to room temperature before use.

Limit Light and Air Exposure

- Light accelerates chemical breakdown; always store oils in a dark place (drawer, cabinet, or box).
- Oxygen causes oxidation, reducing shelf life. Always seal tightly after each use.

Store Upright

- Prevents leakage and reduces the risk of cap degradation or contamination.

Label and Track Shelf Life

- Label bottles with:
    - Name of oil
    - Date of purchase
    - Expiration date (typically 1–3 years depending on the oil)
- Shelf life varies:

- Citrus oils: ~1 year
- Most essential oils: 2–3 years
- Resinous oils (e.g., sandalwood): up to 8 years

Keep Away from Children and Pets

- Essential oils are potent and can be harmful if ingested or misused

Keep Away from Moisture and Contaminants

- Avoid storing oils in bathrooms or humid areas.
- Use clean droppers or pipettes to prevent contamination.

Chapter 4
Methods of usage of Aroma Oil

Inhalation

- Direct inhalation: Add a few drops to a tissue or cotton ball and breathe in gently.
- Steam inhalation: Add 2–3 drops to a bowl of hot water, cover your head with a towel, and inhale the steam.
- Benefits: Clears sinuses, uplifts mood, relieves stress and headaches.

Dry evaporation

- This method only requires some type of dry material, such as a cotton ball or fabric.
- Add a few drops of essential oil to the material. Hold this to your nose and inhale or allow the scent to disperse naturally.
- You can add the material to the vents in your car, your shirt collar, or your pillowcase.

Diffusion

- Electric or ultrasonic diffusers: Mix water and a few drops of oil to disperse aroma into the air.
- Reed diffusers: Use reeds in a bottle of diluted oil for passive scent release.
- Nebulizers: Disperse pure oil without water for stronger effects.
- Benefits: Creates a calming atmosphere, purifies air, supports sleep.

Bath and Shower

- Bath soak: Mix 5–10 drops with a carrier oil (e.g., coconut, jojoba) and add to warm bathwater.
- Shower steam: Drop oil onto the shower floor away from direct water flow.
- Benefits: Relieves muscle tension, enhances relaxation.

Topical Application

- Massage: Blend essential oil with a carrier oil and massage into skin.
- Spot treatment: Apply diluted oil to temples, wrists, or soles of feet.
- Compresses: Add oil to warm or cold compresses for localized relief.
- Benefits: Eases pain, improves circulation, supports skin health.

Household Uses

- Natural cleaning: Add oils like lemon or tea tree to vinegar-based cleaners.
- Linen sprays: Mix oils with water and alcohol for refreshing fabric sprays.
- Pest repellent: Use peppermint or eucalyptus to deter insects.

Emotional and Energetic Uses

- Meditation aid: Use grounding oils like sandalwood or vetiver during mindfulness practice.
- Chakra balancing: Apply diluted oils to pulse points aligned with energy centers (e.g., ylang-ylang for the heart).
- Mood rollers: Create roll-on blends for focus, calm, or confidence using essential oils and fractionated coconut oil.

- Culinary and Edible Uses *(Only with food-grade oils and expert guidance)*
- Flavoring: Add a drop of peppermint or lemon oil to desserts or beverages.
- Herbal infusions: Use oils like basil or rosemary in olive oil for salad dressings.

Caution: Always verify that the oil is labeled GRAS (Generally Recognized As Safe) and use sparingly.

Safety Tips

- Patch test before full use to check for allergies.
- Avoid ingestion unless under professional guidance.
- Keep away from eyes, mucous membranes, and children
- Essential oils have the potential to aggravate the skin. Avoid using essential oils near sensitive areas such as the eyes, ears, and mouth. Do not apply them to broken, inflamed, or irritated skin.
- Always mix essential oils with a therapeutic-grade carrier oil. If you have nut allergies, avoid oils derived from tree nuts.
- Check for potential skin reactions before use. To do a patch test, rub a few drops of diluted essential oil into your inner wrist or below your ear. Wait 24 hours to see if any irritation occurs.
- Certain citrus oils can cause photosensitivity when skin is exposed to sunlight after use. Avoid using any areas of skin that will be exposed to the sun within 12 hours.

- Do not swallow, smoke, or otherwise ingest essential oils. Essential oils are not safe to use internally.
- Talk with a healthcare professional before using essential oils if you take any medications or have an underlying condition, such as high blood pressure, low immunity, or epilepsy.
- People who are pregnant or nursing should also consult with a healthcare professional before use. Essential oils are not recommended for use in children under age 12.

Chapter 5

How Aroma Oil Works

INHALATION

The olfactory nerve (cranial nerve I) is the first and shortest cranial nerve, responsible for your sense of smell. It transmits sensory information from the nasal cavity to the brain's olfactory cortex.

Anatomy of the Olfactory Nerve

- Origin: Arises from the *olfactory epithelium* in the upper part of the nasal cavity.

  Pathway:

- Olfactory receptor neurons send axons through the cribriform plate of the ethmoid bone.
- These axons synapse in the olfactory bulb, which lies just above the nasal cavity.
- Signals then travel via the olfactory tract to the olfactory cortex in the temporal lobe.
- Type: Special visceral afferent (SVA) nerve—transmits sensory data related to smell.

Function

- Detects volatile chemical compounds (odorants) in the air.
- Converts chemical signals into electrical impulses interpreted as smell.

- Plays a role in flavor perception, emotional memory, and danger detection (e.g., smoke, gas).

Unique Features

- Only cranial nerves are exposed to the external environment, making it susceptible to toxins and pathogens.
- Does not pass through the thalamus, unlike other sensory pathways.
- Direct link to limbic system, influencing emotion and memory.

PHYSIOLOGY OF OLFACTORY NERVE

1. Odor Detection

- Odorants (volatile chemical molecules) enter the nasal cavity during breathing or sniffing.
- They dissolve in the mucus layer of the olfactory epithelium, located in the upper nasal cavity.

2. Receptor Activation

- Odorants bind to olfactory receptors on the cilia of olfactory sensory neurons.
- These receptors are G-protein-coupled and trigger a cascade:
- Activation of adenylate cyclase
- Increase in cyclic AMP (cAMP)
- Opening of Na^+ and Ca^{2+} channels
- Depolarization of the neuron

3. Signal Transmission

- Depolarized neurons send action potentials through fila olfactoria (bundles of axons).
- These axons pass through the cribriform plate of the ethmoid bone to reach the olfactory bulb.

4. Central Processing

In the olfactory bulb, axons synapse with mitral and tufted cells in structures called glomeruli.

Signals are relayed via the olfactory tract to:

➔ Primary olfactory cortex (piriform cortex)
➔ Amygdala Land entorhinal cortex (emotion and memory)
➔ Orbitofrontal cortex (conscious odor perception)

5. Unique Features

- No thalamic relay: Unlike other senses, olfactory signals bypass the thalamus initially.
- Neurogenesis: Olfactory neurons regenerate throughout life.
- Direct limbic connection: Explains why smells evoke strong emotions and memories.

Clinical Relevance

- Anosmia: Loss of smell due to trauma, viral infections, neurodegenerative diseases (e.g., Parkinson's, Alzheimer's).

- Testing: Smell identification tests using non-irritating substances (e.g., coffee, vanilla).
- Injury Risk: The nerve is vulnerable to shearing forces in head trauma due to its passage through the cribriform plate.

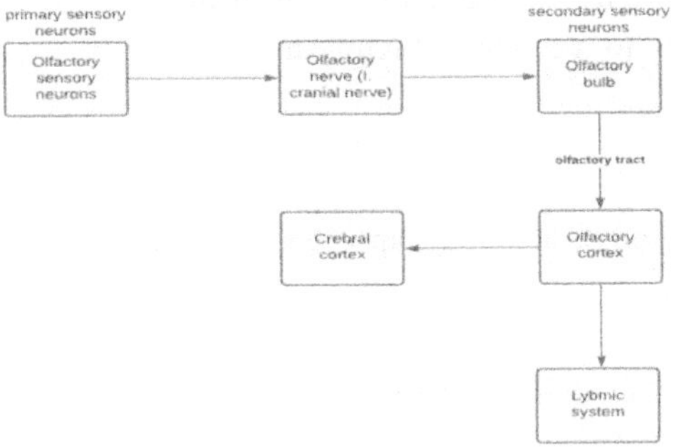

DERMAL ABSORPTION

Essential oils are minute particles where skin is permeable for fat soluble substances and relatively impermeable to water soluble substances.

Absorption also occurs through hair follicles & sweat glads

Rate of circulation and warmth of skin increases the blood flow to surface thereby increases skin's ability to absorb oil

Application of aromatic oil to skin

↓

Oil passes through stratum corneum

↓

Oil molecules passes through dermis

↓

Capillaries

↓

Blood stream

Chapter 6

Fragrance category of Aroma Oil

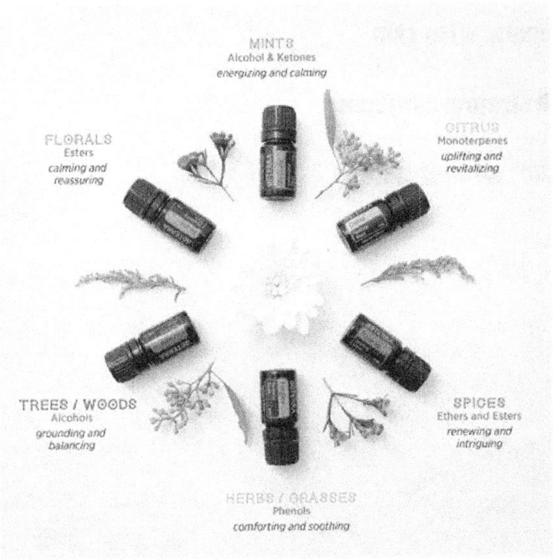

FLORAL

Floral aroma oils are extracted from petals, buds, and sometimes leaves of flowering plants. Their fragrances range from light and powdery to rich and exotic, making them staples in both therapeutic and cosmetic applications.

Oil	Scent Profile	Therapeutic Properties
Lavender	Soft, herbaceous, floral	Calming, sleep-inducing, anti-inflammatory
Rose	Rich, romantic, sweet	Mood-lifting, skin rejuvenating, aphrodisiac
Jasmine	Exotic, warm, sweet	Euphoric, stress-relieving
Ylang ylang	Intense, sweet, tropical	Balancing, sedative, lowers blood pressure
Geranium	Green, rosy, fresh	Hormone-balancing, anti-anxiety, skin toning
Chamomil	Soft, apple-like, gentle	Anti-inflammatory, calming, digestive ai
Tuberose	Rich, creamy, narcotic	Deeply relaxing, aphrodisiac, emotionally grounding
Clary sage	Earthy, herbal-floral	Hormonal support, antidepressant, sedative

Uses of Floral Aroma Oils

- Aromatherapy: Diffused to promote relaxation, emotional balance, and inner peace.
- Skincare: Added to creams and serums for anti-aging and soothing effects.
- Haircare: Used in oils and masks to nourish scalp and promote shine.
- Perfumery: Form the heart notes in many classic and modern fragrances.
- Bath & Body: Infused in bath soaks, body oils, and linen sprays for a luxurious experience.

CITRUS

Citrus aroma oils are known for their fresh, zesty, and uplifting scent profiles. Extracted primarily from the peels of citrus fruits, they are widely used for energizing the mind, purifying the air, and enhancing mood.

Citrus oils belong to the *Rutaceae* family and are typically cold-pressed from fruit rinds. Their volatile compounds—like limonene and citral—contribute to their invigorating aroma and therapeutic potency.

OIL	Scent profile	Therapeutic properties
Lemon	Sharp, clean, bright	Antibacterial, mood-lifting, detoxifying
Orange	Warm, fruity, cheerful	Antidepressant, calming, immune-boosting
Bergamot	Floral-citrus, soft	Stress-relieving, skin-soothing, emotionally balancing
Grapefruit	Tart, fresh, crisp	Fatigue-reducing, appetite-suppressing, cleansing
Lime	Tangy, green, vibrant	Refreshing, antiseptic, mentally stimulating
Mandarin	Sweet, gentle, child-friendly	Digestive aid, calming, skin-friendly
Yuzu	Complex, lemony-floral	Anti-inflammatory, uplifting, exotic aroma

Uses of Citrus Aroma Oils

- Aromatherapy: Diffused to boost energy, reduce stress, and purify indoor air.
- Skincare: Added to toners and masks for brightening and antibacterial effects (use with caution—some are photosensitive).
- Cleaning: Used in natural cleaners for their antimicrobial and deodorizing properties.
- Perfumery: Common top notes in fresh and fruity fragrance blends.
- Mood Support: Ideal for morning routines, workspaces, and emotional reset.

WOODY

Woody aroma oils are known for their earthy, grounding, and warm scent profiles. They evoke a sense of stability, calm, and connection to nature, making them ideal for meditation, stress relief, and masculine fragrance blends.

Woody oils are typically extracted from bark, roots, resins, and heartwood of trees. Their deep, dry, and sometimes smoky notes form the base of many perfumes and therapeutic blends. These oils are prized for their longevity and emotional depth.

Oil	Scent profile	Therapeutic properties
Sandalwood	Creamy, soft, sweet-woody	Calming, meditative, anti-inflammatory, aphrodisiac
Cedarwood	Dry, balsamic, forest-like	Calming, meditative, anti-inflammatory, aphrodisiac
Patchouli	Earthy, musky, rich	Mood-balancing, skin-healing, sensual
Vetiver	Smoky, earthy, rooty	Deeply relaxing, cooling, stabilizing for emotions
Frankincense	Resinous, woody-citrus	Spiritual, anti-inflammatory, immune-boosting
Oudh (Agarwood)	Exotic, smoky, luxurious	Spiritual elevation, emotional depth, rare and prized in perfumery
Pine	Sharp, fresh, foresty	Respiratory support, energizing, cleansing
Juniper	Crisp, green-woody	Detoxifying, purifying, stress-reducing

Uses of Woody Aroma Oils

- Aromatherapy: Used in diffusers to promote tranquility, focus, and emotional grounding.
- Perfumery: Form the base notes in many luxury and masculine fragrances.
- Skincare: Added to serums and balms for anti-aging and anti-inflammatory effects.
- Spiritual Practice: Incorporated into rituals, meditation, and incense for sacred ambiance.

- Home Fragrance: Ideal for cozy, warm, and forest-inspired atmospheres.

HERBAL / GREEN

Herbal/Green aroma oils are fresh, crisp, and invigorating, often evoking the scent of leaves, stems, and garden herbs. They are prized for their clarifying, cooling, and purifying properties—ideal for mental focus, respiratory support, and emotional refreshment.

These oils are typically steam-distilled from herbs, grasses, and foliage. Their scent profiles range from minty and camphorous to leafy and slightly bitter.

Oil	Scent profile	Therapeutic indications
Peppermint	Sharp, minty, cooling	Mental clarity, headache relief, digestive aid
Eucalyptus	Camphorous, fresh, sharp	Respiratory support, antimicrobial, energizing
Basil	Sweet-herbal, spicy	Anti-inflammatory, mental focus, stress relief
Thyme	Strong, earthy, medicinal	Immune-boosting, antibacterial, warming

Rosemary	Herbaceous, pine-like	Memory-enhancing, circulation-boosting, hair growth
Tea Tree	Medicinal, green, pungent	Antiseptic, acne-fighting, immune support
Lemongrass	Citrusy-green, sharp	Purifying, insect-repelling, muscle-relaxing
Spearmint	Sweet-minty, gentle	Mood-lifting, digestive aid, child-friendly alternative to peppermint
Bay Leaf	Spicy-green, woody	Pain relief, respiratory support, grounding

Uses of Herbal/Green Aroma Oils

- Aromatherapy: Diffused for mental clarity, respiratory ease, and emotional refreshment.
- Skincare: Used in toners and acne treatments for their antibacterial and anti-inflammatory effects.
- Haircare: Added to oils and shampoos to stimulate growth and reduce dandruff.
- Cleaning: Incorporated into natural disinfectants and air purifiers.
- Massage & Bath: Blended for muscle relief and circulation support.

SPICY

Spicy aroma oils are bold, warm, and invigorating—often used to stimulate circulation, energize the senses, and add depth to seasonal blends. They're especially popular in autumn and winter for their comforting and exotic character.

Spicy oils are typically steam-distilled or cold-pressed from seeds, barks, and roots of aromatic spices. Their scent profiles range from sweet and fiery to dry and peppery, making them ideal for both therapeutic and perfumery applications.

Oil	Scent profile	Therapeutic indication
Clove	Warm, sweet, pungent	Antiseptic, pain-relieving, emotionally warming
Cinnamon Bark	Sweet, spicy, intense	Circulation-boosting, aphrodisiac, immune-enhancing
Ginger	Sharp, earthy, peppery	Digestive aid, anti-nausea, energizing
Cardamom	Sweet, balsamic, exotic	Mood-lifting, respiratory support, sensual
Nutmeg	Warm, nutty, slightly sweet	Sedative, anti-inflammatory, comforting
Black pepper	Dry, sharp, woody-spicy	Stimulating, detoxifying, muscle-relieving
allspice	Complex, clove-like	Uplifting, warming, emotionally grounding
Bay leaf	Spicy-green, woody	Respiratory support, pain relief, grounding

Uses of Spicy Aroma Oils

- Aromatherapy: Diffused to energize, warm, and uplift mood—especially in colder seasons.
- Massage & Bath: Blended for muscle relief and circulation support (use diluted).
- Perfumery: Adds depth and warmth to oriental and gourmand fragrance profiles.
- Home Fragrance: Popular in festive blends, potpourri, and seasonal room sprays.
- Culinary & Medicinal: Some (like clove and ginger) are used in herbal remedies and flavoring.

Chapter 7
Essential Oils

7.1 Amrette Seed Essential Oil (Ambrette Seed Oil)

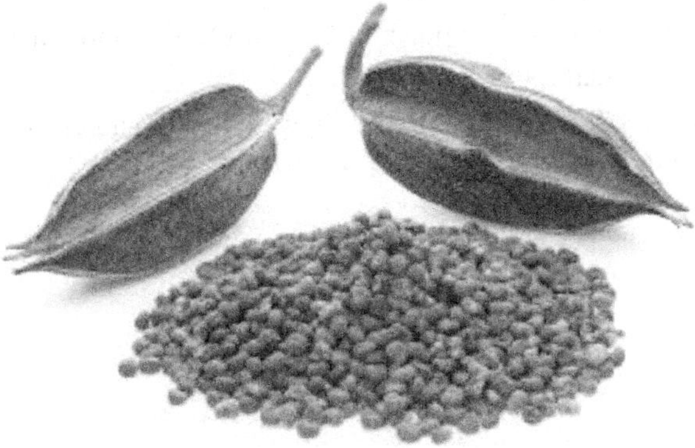

Introduction

Amrette Seed essential Oil, also known as Ambrette Seed Oil, is a rare and luxurious oil extracted from the seeds of the Abelmoschus moschatus plant, commonly called musk mallow. Native to India and other tropical regions, the plant has been valued for centuries for its aromatic and medicinal properties.

This oil is renowned for its rich, musky, and slightly floral aroma, making it a prized ingredient in natural perfumery as a botanical alternative to animal-derived musk. In addition to its exquisite fragrance, Amrette Seed Essential Oil is used in aromatherapy, skincare, and traditional medicine for its calming, aphrodisiac, and anti-inflammatory qualities.

Its unique composition, especially the presence of ambrettolide, gives it a deep and sensual scent that lingers, making it a sought-after base note and fixative in high-end perfumes and essential oil blends.

Botanical Information

- Botanical Name: *Abelmoschus moschatus*
- Family: Malvaceae
- Common Names: Musk mallow, Ambrette seed, Musk seed
- Plant Part Used: Seeds
- Extraction Method: Steam distillation or solvent extraction of dried seeds
- Origin: Native to India; cultivated in tropical regions like Indonesia, China, and the West Indies

Chemical Composition

Ambrette seed oil contains several aromatic compounds. Key constituents include:

- Ambrettolide (macrocyclic lactone) – provides a musky aroma
- Farnesol – floral scent
- Musk ambrette
- Myristic acid
- Palmitic acid
- β-Caryophyllene – anti-inflammatory
- Linalool – soothing scent

- Geraniol – rose-like aroma

Note: Composition can vary based on climate, soil, and extraction method.

Uses and Applications

Aromatherapy

- Uplifts mood
- Reduces stress and anxiety
- Calms the nervous system
- Promotes emotional balance

Perfumery

- Fixative in perfumes (holds scent longer)
- Adds depth and warmth to floral and oriental perfumes
- Used in both **masculine and feminine fragrances**

Cosmetics & Skincare

- Adds fragrance to lotions, creams, and soaps
- Contains antioxidant and antimicrobial properties
- May help tone and nourish skin (when diluted)

Traditional Medicine (Ayurveda & Unani)

- Used to treat **cramps, digestive issues, and nervous disorders**
- Believed to act as an **aphrodisiac**
- Sometimes used for **cough, cold, and asthma**

Massage Therapy

- Blended with carrier oils for muscle relaxation
- Soothes joint pain and inflammation

Safety and Precautions

- Always dilute before topical application (e.g., with jojoba or coconut oil)
- Perform a patch test to avoid allergic reactions
- Avoid during pregnancy or breastfeeding
- Not recommended for internal use
- Store in a cool, dark place

Sustainability and Ethics

- Often considered more ethical than animal musk (from musk deer)
- Plant-derived and biodegradable
- Organic and wildcrafted sources are available

Summary of Benefits

Benefit	Description
Natural Musk Scent	Excellent fixative for perfumes
Mood Enhancement	Calms nerves, reduces anxiety

Skin Benefits	Toning, anti-inflammatory, aromatic use in skincare
Aphrodisiac	Traditionally used to enhance libido
Respiratory Support	Helps with cough and asthma (inhaling or topical use)

7.2 Aniseed essential oil

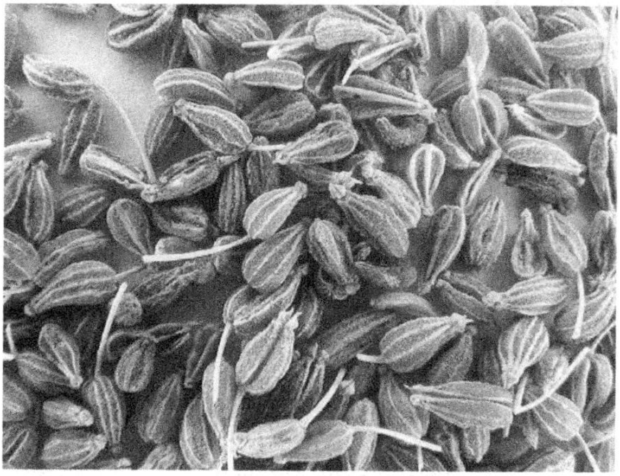

Aniseed essential oil is a sweet, licorice-scented oil derived from the seeds of the anise plant (*Pimpinella anisum*), a flowering herb native to the Mediterranean and Southwest Asia. It has been traditionally valued for centuries in Greek, Roman, and Ayurvedic medicine for its powerful effects on digestion, respiratory health, and hormonal balance.

The oil is typically extracted through steam distillation of the dried seeds and contains a high percentage of anethole, the compound responsible for its characteristic aroma and therapeutic properties. Aniseed essential oil is known for being carminative, antispasmodic, expectorant, and mildly estrogenic.

Botanical Information

- Common Name: Anise, Aniseed
- Botanical Name: *Pimpinella anisum*
- Family: Apiaceae (Umbelliferae – carrot or parsley family)

- Part Used: Seeds (fruits)
- Extraction Method: Steam distillation
- Origin: Native to the eastern Mediterranean and Southwest Asia
- Color: Colorless to pale yellow
- Aroma: Sweet, spicy, warm, licorice-like

Major Chemical Constituents

Compound	Function
Anethole (80–90%)	Antispasmodic, carminative, expectorant
Estragole (Methyl chavicol)	Antioxidant, stimulant
Limonene	Antimicrobial, uplifting
α-Pinene & β-Pinene	Antiseptic, anti-inflammatory

Note: Anethole is the key active compound responsible for the oil's distinct licorice scent and medicinal actions.

Therapeutic Properties

- Antispasmodic
- Carminative (relieves gas and bloating)
- Expectorant (clears mucus)
- Estrogenic (mimics estrogen activity)
- Antiseptic
- Digestive stimulant
- Sedative (mild)

- Insecticidal

Aromatherapy & Emotional Effects

- Soothing and calming: May relieve stress, nervous tension, and mild depression
- Uplifting: Acts as a mild mood booster
- Mental clarity: Promotes focus when used in small amounts Aromatherapy Diffuser Blend (for focus & clarity):
- 2 drops Aniseed
- 3 drops Sweet Orange
- 2 drops Rosemary

Topical & Internal Uses

Use diluted (at 1% or less) for topical application. Internal use should only be done under the guidance of a qualified professional.

- For indigestion, cramps, or bloating: Rub diluted oil on the abdomen in circular motions
- For respiratory relief: Use in steam inhalation to loosen mucus and soothe cough
- For menstrual discomfort: Apply to lower abdomen to ease spasms

Household & Culinary Uses

- Acts as a natural insect repellent
- Used to flavor liqueurs (e.g., ouzo, sambuca, absinthe)
- Occasionally added in natural toothpaste or mouthwashes

- Can freshen air when diffused, especially in wintertime blends

Traditional & Historical Uses

- Used in Ancient Egypt, Greece, and Rome for digestion and breath freshening
- Common in Ayurvedic and Unani medicine for its warming and digestive qualities
- Traditionally used to stimulate lactation (though now used with caution)

Safety and Precautions

- Avoid during pregnancy and breastfeeding due to estrogenic effects
- Avoid in cases of estrogen-sensitive conditions (like breast cancer)
- Use in low dilutions: Anethole can be a skin and mucous membrane irritant
- Not recommended for infants or young children
- Avoid long-term use: May cause sensitization or toxicity with overuse

Storage

- Store in a cool, dry place, away from sunlight
- Shelf life: Approximately 2–3 years
- Always keep tightly sealed

7.3 Angelica Essential Oil

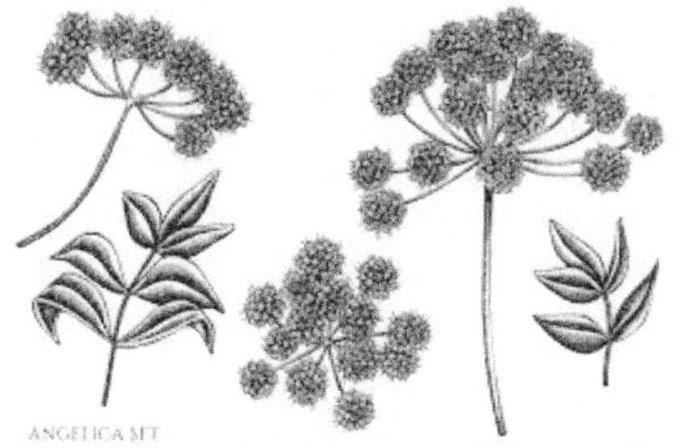

Angelica Essential Oil is a highly valued aromatic oil obtained mainly from the roots of *Angelica archangelica*, a biennial herb belonging to the Apiaceae family. It is native to Europe and parts of Asia and has been traditionally used in herbal medicine for centuries.

Botanical Information

- Botanical name: *Angelica archangelica*
- Family: Apiaceae (Umbelliferae)
- Common names: Garden Angelica, European Angelica, Wild Celery
- Part used: Root (main), seeds
- Origin: Europe (especially France, Germany), also cultivated in India and Scandinavia
- Extraction method: Steam distillation
- Oil yield: Approximately 0.3–1%

Physical & Chemical Properties

- Color: Pale yellow to amber
- Odor: Earthy, woody, musky, slightly peppery
- Consistency: Medium
- Perfumery note: Base to middle note
- Main chemical constituents:
    - α-Pinene
    - β-Pinene
    - Limonene
    - Linalool
    - Furanocoumarins (especially in root oil)

Therapeutic Properties

- Carminative – Relieves gas and bloating
- Digestive stimulant – Improves appetite and digestion
- Expectorant – Helps remove mucus in respiratory conditions
- Diaphoretic – Promotes sweating
- Antispasmodic – Relieves muscle cramps
- Calming (mild sedative) – Reduces nervous tension
- Detoxifying – Supports lymphatic drainage

Therapeutic Uses

Digestive System

- Indigestion
- Flatulence
- Loss of appetite
- Colic

Respiratory System

- Bronchitis
- Cough

- Cold
- Congestion

Musculoskeletal System

- Rheumatism
- Arthritis
- Muscle pain

Nervous System

- Stress
- Anxiety
- Fatigue
- Emotional exhaustion

Aromatherapy Applications

- Diffusion: For stress, respiratory congestion
- Massage oil: 1–2% dilution for muscle pain & digestive massage
- Steam inhalation: For cough and bronchitis
- Bath: For detoxification and fatigue

Safety & Precautions

- Phototoxic: Due to furanocoumarins (avoid sun exposure after topical application)
- Avoid during pregnancy
- Avoid in diabetes (may affect blood sugar)
- Always dilute before skin use (1–2%)
- Perform patch test

Blending with Other Oils

Angelica blends well with:

- Bergamot
- Lavender
- Clary Sage

- Patchouli
- Sandalwood
- Cedarwood

7.4 Basil essential Oil

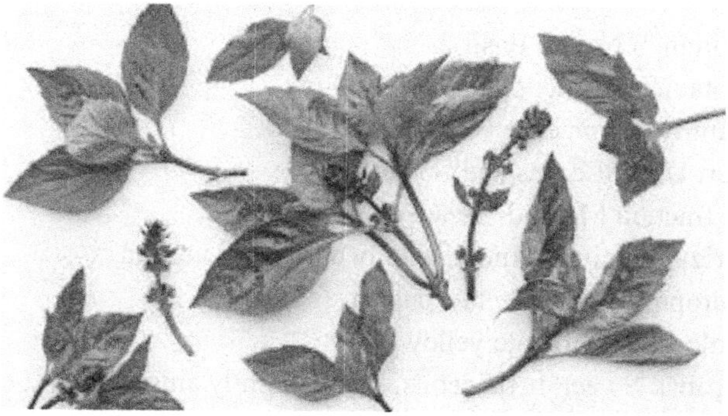

Introduction

Basil essential oil is a highly aromatic and therapeutic oil extracted from the leaves and flowering tops of the *Ocimum basilicum* plant, a member of the mint (Lamiaceae) family. Native to India and other tropical regions of Asia, basil has been used for centuries in Ayurvedic, Greek, and Roman medicine for its healing, culinary, and spiritual properties.

The essential oil is most commonly obtained through steam distillation and is known for its sweet, herbaceous, and slightly spicy aroma. It contains powerful compounds like linalool, eugenol, and methyl chavicol, which give it antibacterial, anti-inflammatory, antispasmodic, and nervine (nerve-calming) properties.

Basil essential oil is widely used in aromatherapy to ease mental fatigue, anxiety, and headaches, and also in topical applications to support the muscles, joints, and digestive system. Its refreshing scent and therapeutic effects make it a versatile oil in natural health and wellness practices.

Botanical Information

- Common Name: Basil
- Botanical Name: *Ocimum basilicum*
- Family: Lamiaceae (mint family)
- Part Used: Leaves and flowering tops
- Extraction Method: Steam distillation
- Origin: Native to India, widely cultivated in Asia, Europe, and the Mediterranean
- Color: Clear to pale yellow
- Aroma: Sweet, herbaceous, spicy, slightly anise-like

Major Chemical Constituents

Compound	Function
Linalool	Calming, anti-inflammatory, skin-friendly
Methyl chavicol (Estragole)	Stimulating, antispasmodic, digestive aid
Eugenol	Antiseptic, anesthetic, anti-inflammatory
Cineole (1,8-cineole)	Expectorant, respiratory support
Ocimene & Camphene	Antioxidant, antibacterial

Note: The chemical makeup can vary by basil type (sweet basil, holy basil, lemon basil, etc.)

Therapeutic Properties

- Antibacterial
- Antiviral
- Antifungal
- Anti-inflammatory
- Antispasmodic
- Analgesic
- Nervine (strengthens the nervous system)
- Carminative (relieves gas)
- Expectorant

Aromatherapy & Emotional Benefits

- Reduces mental fatigue, headaches, and anxiety
- Improves focus, concentration, and clarity
- Used in meditation to stimulate the mind and calm the nerves

Diffuser Blend for Focus:

- 3 drops Basil
- 2 drops Lemon
- 2 drops Rosemary

Topical Uses

Always dilute with a carrier oil (like jojoba, almond, or coconut oil)

- Muscle tension & cramps: Apply to affected areas
- Acne or skin infections: Antibacterial action helps reduce breakouts
- Headache relief: Apply diluted oil to temples or back of the neck

- Insect bites: Reduces inflammation and itching

Household & Practical Uses

- Acts as a natural insect repellent
- Used in herbal sprays to purify the air
- Added to massage blends for relaxation and circulation

Traditional & Ayurvedic Uses

- Known as "Tulsi" in India (though true Tulsi is *Ocimum sanctum*)
- Used in Ayurveda for respiratory disorders, digestion, and mental clarity
- Employed in herbal teas, tonics, and poultices for inflammation and infections

Safety and Precautions

- Dilution is essential: Basil oil can irritate sensitive skin
- Pregnancy/Nursing: Use cautiously (especially varieties high in estragole)
- Avoid on young children: May be too stimulating
- Contraindicated in epilepsy: Due to its stimulant properties
- Short-term use recommended: Prolonged exposure can lead to sensitization

Storage

- Store in a cool, dark place
- Keep tightly sealed
- Shelf life: About 2–3 years if stored properly

7.5 Bergamot essential Oil

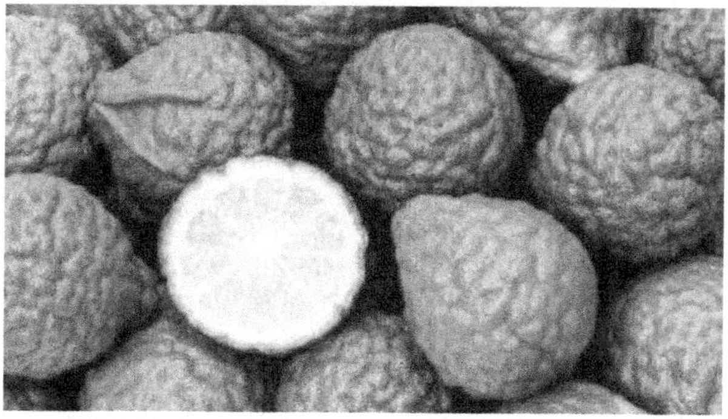

Introduction

Bergamot essential oil is a refreshing and uplifting citrus oil extracted from the rind of the bergamot orange (*Citrus bergamia*), a small fruit resembling a cross between an orange and a lime. Native to Southern Italy, particularly the Calabria region, bergamot has been prized for centuries in traditional medicine, perfumery, and tea flavoring—most famously in Earl Grey tea.

The oil is typically obtained through cold expression of the fruit peel and is cherished for its fresh, sweet, slightly floral aroma with subtle spicy undertones. It contains active constituents like limonene, linalool, and linalyl acetate, which give it powerful antidepressant, antibacterial, anti-inflammatory, and calming properties.

In aromatherapy, bergamot is often used to reduce stress, uplift the mood, and promote relaxation, making it a popular choice for emotional balance and mental clarity. However, due to its phototoxicity (when cold-pressed), it must be used with care on the skin unless labeled FCF (furanocoumarin-free).

Botanical Information

- Common Name: Bergamot
- Botanical Name: *Citrus bergamia*
- Family: Rutaceae (citrus family)
- Part Used: Rind (peel) of the fruit
- Extraction Method: Cold expression (sometimes steam distilled)
- Origin: Native to Southern Italy; also grown in Ivory Coast, Morocco, and Argentina
- Color: Green to yellow-green
- Aroma: Fresh, sweet, citrusy with floral and slightly spicy undertones

Major Chemical Constituents

Compound	Function
Limonene	Uplifting, antibacterial, cleansing
Linalyl acetate	Relaxing, soothing, sedative
Linalool	Antiseptic, calming, skin-healing
Bergapten *(only in cold-pressed oil)*	Phototoxic agent, UV-sensitive
α-Pinene & β-Pinene	Antiseptic, decongestant
Terpineol	Anti-inflammatory, mild sedative

Note: The presence of bergapten makes cold-pressed bergamot oil phototoxic. FCF (furanocoumarin-free) versions are available and safer for skin use.

Therapeutic Properties

- Antidepressant
- Anxiolytic (reduces anxiety)
- Antiseptic
- Analgesic
- Antispasmodic
- Digestive stimulant
- Deodorant
- Sedative
- Cicatrizant (promotes wound healing)

Aromatherapy & Emotional Benefits

- Calms nervous tension, anxiety, and stress-related conditions
- Eases mild depression and promotes emotional balance
- Improves sleep and reduces agitation
- Uplifts mood while grounding the mind

Diffuser Blend for Calm & Clarity:

- 3 drops Bergamot
- 2 drops Lavender
- 2 drops Frankincense

Topical Applications

Dilute to 1–2% and avoid direct sunlight after use unless it's FCF (bergapten-free).

- For acne and oily skin: Acts as a natural astringent and cleanser
- For eczema or psoriasis: Soothes irritation and supports skin regeneration
- Massage oil for stress relief: Blended with carrier oils like jojoba or sweet almond
- Deodorant and perfume base: Fresh citrusy fragrance with staying power

Internal and Culinary Uses

Only under supervised, therapeutic-grade applications – not recommended for casual internal use.

- Used in Earl Grey tea as flavoring
- Occasional use in culinary desserts and flavorings

Household Uses

- Natural air freshener and diffuser oil
- Deodorizes spaces while providing emotional uplift
- Can be added to homemade surface sprays

Traditional & Cultural Uses

- Long used in Italian folk medicine for fever, parasites, and skin conditions
- Used in traditional perfumery (especially colognes) for centuries
- Ingredient in Aromatherapie Classique for mood balance

Safety & Precautions

- Phototoxicity: Cold-pressed bergamot contains bergapten, which can cause severe burns and skin damage when exposed to sunlight/UV rays.
  → Use FCF (furanocoumarin-free) bergamot oil for safe topical use
- Dilution essential: Recommended maximum dermal use level = 0.4% (if not FCF)
- Avoid during pregnancy: In high concentrations
- Avoid use in babies and small children

Storage

- Store in a cool, dark, airtight container
- Sensitive to oxidation – refrigerate to prolong shelf life
- Shelf life: About 1–2 years once opened

7.6 Black Pepper Essential Oil

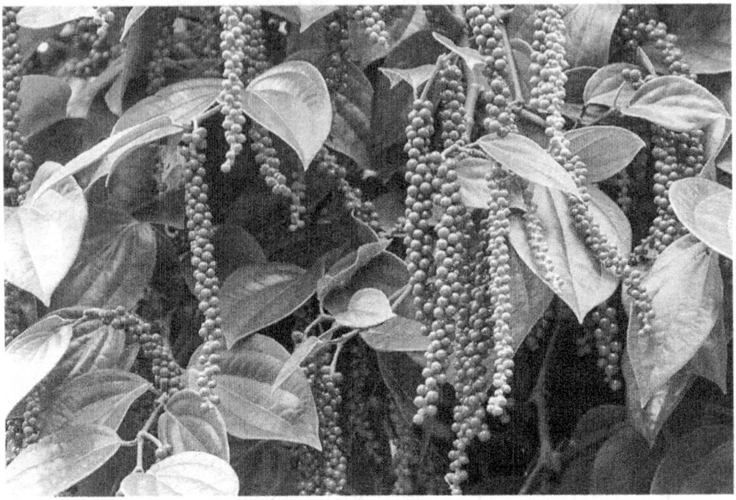

Introduction

Black Pepper Essential Oil is derived from the dried fruit (peppercorns) of the Piper nigrum plant through steam distillation. Known as the "King of Spices", black pepper has been prized for centuries for its flavor, medicinal value, and warming properties. The essential oil has a spicy, warm, woody aroma and is often used in aromatherapy, massage, and natural medicine.

Botanical Information

- Botanical name: *Piper nigrum*
- Family: Piperaceae
- Plant part used: Dried peppercorns (fruit)
- Extraction method: Steam Distillation
- Appearance: Pale yellow to greenish
- Aroma: Warm, spicy, sharp, woody

CHEMICAL COMPOSITION (Main Constituents)

- β-Caryophyllene
- Limonene
- Pinene (α and β)
- Sabinene
- Linalool
- Myrcene

These compounds contribute to its analgesic, anti-inflammatory, and antioxidant properties.

Therapeutic Properties

- Analgesic (pain relief)
- Antispasmodic
- Anti-inflammatory
- Antioxidant
- Digestive stimulant
- Circulatory stimulant
- Antibacterial
- Carminative (relieves gas)

Benefits Of Black Pepper Essential Oil

Pain & Muscle Relief

- Helps ease arthritis, muscle cramps, stiffness, and body aches
- Useful in sports massage oils

Improves Digestion

- Stimulates digestive enzymes
- Reduces bloating, gas, and indigestion

Enhances Circulation

- Stimulates blood flow and reduces feelings of coldness or numbness
- Good for detox and lymphatic drainage

Respiratory Relief

- Assists in clearing congestion, cough, and sinusitis
- Can be used in steam inhalation\

Boosts Mental Clarity

- Uplifting and focusing
- Helps relieve mental fatigue and low mood

Detoxification Support

- Encourages sweating and urination, aiding in toxin removal

Antioxidant Protection

- Helps neutralize free radicals
- Protects skin and body from oxidative stress

Uses Of Black Pepper Essential Oil

Aromatherapy:

- Diffuse to stimulate the mind and improve mood

Massage:

- Dilute with a carrier oil to soothe sore muscles and joints

Topical Application:

- Applied (diluted) on the abdomen for digestive support

Inhalation:

- For clearing nasal passages and supporting respiratory health

Blends Well With:

- Bergamot
- Lemon
- Frankincense
- Clove
- Lavender
- Rosemary
- Ginger

PRECAUTIONS

- Always dilute before topical use (2–3% dilution is safe)
- Avoid contact with eyes and mucous membranes
- Not recommended for children under 5 or pregnant women without professional guidance
- May cause skin irritation in sensitive individuals
- Avoid internal use unless under medical supervision

INTERESTING FACTS

- In ancient times, black pepper was used as currency and considered more valuable than gold.
- In traditional medicine (like Ayurveda), it's used to ignite *Agni* (digestive fire).

7.7 Camphor essential oil

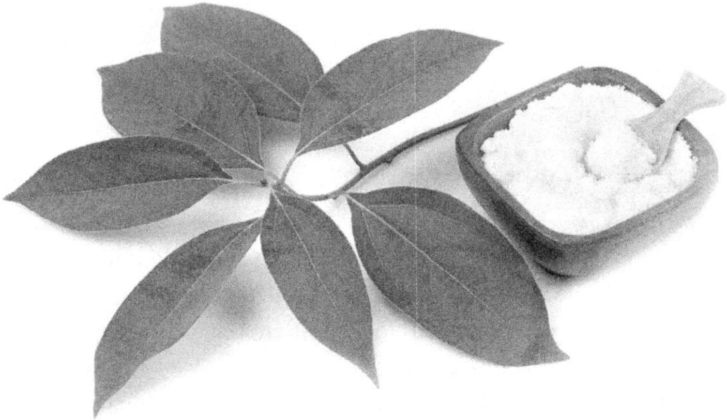

Introduction

Camphor essential oil is derived from the wood of the Camphor tree (*Cinnamomum camphora*), which is native to Asia, particularly Japan, China, and Taiwan. This oil has been used for centuries in traditional medicine for its cooling, anti-inflammatory, and stimulant properties.

There are three types of camphor oil based on chemical composition:

- White camphor oil (safe and most commonly used in aromatherapy)
- Brown camphor oil (toxic; not used therapeutically)
- Yellow camphor oil (also considered toxic)

Only white camphor oil is safe for external use.

Botanical Information

- Botanical name: *Cinnamomum camphora*
- Family: Lauraceae
- Plant part used: Wood, bark
- Extraction method: Steam Distillation
- Appearance: Colorless or pale yellow
- Aroma: Sharp, penetrating, clean, medicinal

Chemical Constituents (White Camphor Oil)

- 1,8-Cineole (Eucalyptol)
- Camphor
- Borneol
- Pinene
- Terpineol
- Limonene

These compounds are responsible for its cooling, decongestant, and stimulant effects.

Therapeutic Properties

- Analgesic (pain-relieving)
- Antiseptic
- Anti-inflammatory
- Decongestant
- Antispasmodic
- Stimulant
- Insect repellent
- Antimicrobial

Benefits Of Camphor Essential Oil

Relieves Cough and Congestion

- Acts as a decongestant and expectorant
- Used in vaporizers and chest rubs for colds, flu, bronchitis

Soothes Muscle Pain and Cramps

- Relieves arthritis, muscle stiffness, and joint pain
- Cooling sensation reduces inflammation

Improves Circulation

- Stimulates blood flow
- Eases swelling and inflammation

Skin Conditions

- Useful for itchiness, eczema, acne, and fungal infections
- Antiseptic properties prevent skin infections

Stress and Anxiety Relief

- Mild sedative and nervine
- Calms nerves, relieves fatigue and nervous tension

Insect Repellent

- Natural repellent against mosquitoes, flies, and mites

Uses of Camphor Essential Oil

Aromatherapy:

- Used in diffusers to clear the sinuses and refresh the air

Topical Use (Diluted):

- Mixed with a carrier oil and applied to painful areas
- Included in balms and ointments

Steam Inhalation:

- Clears blocked nasal passages

Blends Well With:

- Eucalyptus
- Rosemary
- Lavender
- Peppermint
- Basil
- Cajeput

Precautions

- Use only white camphor oil – brown and yellow camphor oils are toxic
- Always dilute before applying to skin (1–2% dilution)
- Do not ingest; can be toxic if swallowed
- Avoid during pregnancy and for young children
- May trigger seizures in some individuals if used in high amounts
- Avoid contact with eyes, mucous membranes, and open wounds

Interesting Facts

- In traditional Chinese and Indian medicine, camphor has been used for centuries as a cooling remedy.
- It was once used as an embalming agent due to its strong antiseptic properties.
- Commonly found in Vicks VapoRub, balms, ointments, and cooling gels.

7.8 Cardamom Essential Oil

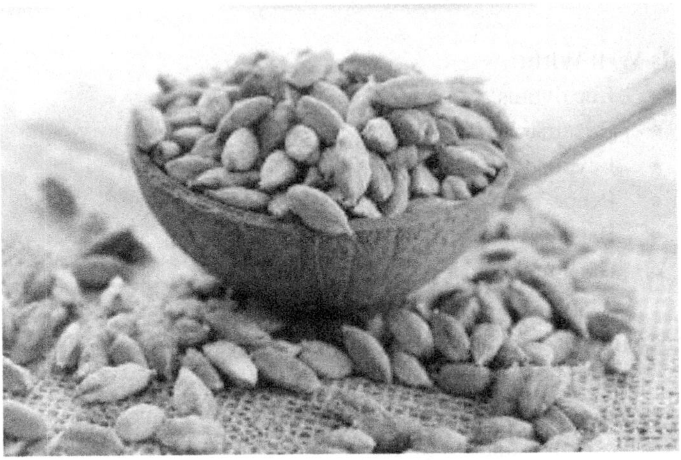

Introduction

Cardamom Essential Oil is extracted from the seeds of the Elettaria cardamomum plant, a perennial herb native to India and Sri Lanka. Known as the "Queen of Spices," cardamom has been widely used in Ayurveda, Unani, and traditional Chinese medicine for its therapeutic benefits.

Its oil has a sweet, spicy, and slightly woody aroma and is highly valued for its ability to aid digestion, uplift mood, and support respiratory health.

Botanical Information

- BOTANICAL NAME: *Elettaria cardamomum*
- FAMILY: Zingiberaceae (Ginger family)
- PLANT PART USED: Seeds (pods)
- EXTRACTION METHOD: Steam Distillation
- APPEARANCE: Clear to pale yellow

- AROMA: Warm, sweet, spicy, balsamic
-

Chemical Composition (Major Components)

- Cineole (1,8-Cineole)
- α-Terpinyl acetate
- Limonene
- Linalool
- Myrcene
- Sabinene

These constituents provide its antimicrobial, digestive, and anti-inflammatory effects.

Therapeutic Properties

- Carminative (relieves gas)
- Digestive stimulant
- Antispasmodic
- Expectorant
- Antibacterial
- Aphrodisiac
- Mood enhancer
- Anti-inflammatory
- Antioxidant

Benefits Of Cardamom Essential Oil

1. Digestive Aid

- Eases bloating, gas, indigestion, and nausea
- Stimulates the secretion of gastric juices

2. Respiratory Relief

- Helps relieve coughs, asthma, bronchitis, and congestion
- Acts as a natural expectorant

3. Mental Clarity and Upliftment

- Uplifts mood and helps relieve mental fatigue, stress, and depression
- Enhances focus and alertness

4. Antimicrobial Support

- Fights off oral infections, bad breath, and bacteria
- Used in mouthwashes and toothpaste

5. Aphrodisiac Properties

- Traditionally used to stimulate libido and balance reproductive health

6. Skin Health

- Soothes irritated or inflamed skin
- Helps balance oil production when used in diluted form

Uses of Cardamom Essential Oil

Aromatherapy:

- Diffused to enhance clarity, lift mood, and soothe the respiratory system

Massage Oil:

- Diluted with carrier oils to ease digestion and muscle tension

Topical Use (Diluted):

- Applied on the abdomen for digestive support
- Used in skincare blends for calming effects

Inhalation:

- Clears congestion and supports breathing

Blends Well With:

- Ginger
- Clove
- Orange
- Cinnamon
- Bergamot
- Ylang Ylang
- Cedarwood

Precautions

- Always dilute with a carrier oil before applying to skin (2–3% dilution)
- Avoid use near eyes, nose, or sensitive areas
- Not recommended for pregnant or lactating women without consulting a healthcare provider
- Do not ingest unless prescribed by a qualified professional
- Patch test before use to avoid allergic reaction

Interesting Facts

- Cardamom is one of the oldest known spices, used in Egypt as early as 1500 BC.
- In Ayurveda, it is used to balance Kapha and Vata doshas.
- Cardamom pods were once chewed to sweeten the breath and stimulate digestion.

7.9 Chamomile Essential Oil

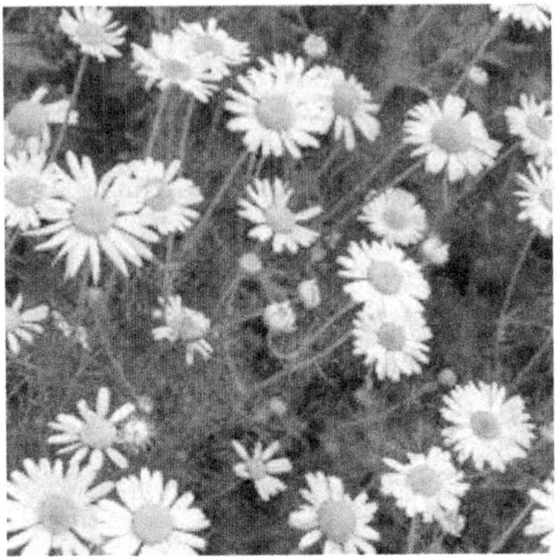

Introduction

Chamomile Essential Oil is extracted from the flowers of Chamomile plants, primarily German Chamomile (*Matricaria chamomilla*) and Roman Chamomile (*Chamaemelum nobile*). It is known for its soothing, calming, anti-inflammatory, and skin-healing properties. With a soft, sweet, and apple-like aroma, chamomile oil has been used since ancient times in Greek, Roman, and Egyptian medicine.

There are two main types of chamomile oil used therapeutically:

Type	Botanical Name	Color	Aroma	Key Benefit
Roman Chamomile	Chamaemelum nobile	Pale yellow	Sweet, fruity, apple-like	Calming & anti-anxiety
German Chamomile	Matricaria chamomilla	Deep blue	Stronger, herbaceous	Anti-inflammatory & skin healing

Botanical Information

- *Chamaemelum nobile* (Roman)
- *Matricaria chamomilla* (German)
- FAMILY: Asteraceae (Daisy family)
- PLANT PART USED: Flower heads
- EXTRACTION METHOD: Steam Distillation
- APPEARANCE: Roman – pale yellow; German – deep blue
- AROMA: Sweet, apple-like, herbaceous

Chemical Composition

- German Chamomile: Chamazulene, α-bisabolol, Bisabolol oxides, Farnesene
- Roman Chamomile: Isobutyl angelate, Anthemic acid, Pinocarvone, Limonene

Therapeutic Properties

- Anti-inflammatory
- Analgesic (pain-relieving)
- Antispasmodic
- Calming & sedative
- Antiseptic
- Antiallergenic
- Antibacterial
- Carminative (gas relief)
- Skin regenerative

Benefits Of Chamomile Essential Oil

1. Reduces Stress & Anxiety

- Promotes relaxation and emotional balance
- Helps treat insomnia, nervous tension, and irritability

2. Soothes Skin Conditions

- Effective against eczema, rashes, dermatitis, acne, and psoriasis
- Accelerates wound healing and reduces skin irritation

3. Relieves Pain & Inflammation

- Helpful in arthritis, muscle pain, joint pain, and menstrual cramps

4. Aids Digestion

- Reduces indigestion, gas, cramping, and nausea

5. Calms Children

- Safe (in diluted form) for treating teething pain, colic, and hyperactivity in children

6. Promotes Better Sleep

- Natural sedative; diffusing before bedtime supports deep sleep

Uses of Chamomile Essential Oil

Aromatherapy:

- Diffuse to relieve anxiety and induce calmness

Topical Application:

- Diluted in carrier oil and applied to skin for anti-inflammatory and soothing effects

Bath Soak:

- Add a few drops to warm bathwater to calm the body and mind

Massage:

- Used in massage oils for cramps, pain, and emotional tension

Blends Well With:

- Lavender
- Rose
- Geranium
- Ylang Ylang
- Clary Sage
- Bergamot

Precautions

- Always dilute before applying to skin (1–2%)
- Perform a patch test to rule out allergic reactions, especially for people allergic to ragweed or daisies
- Not recommended for pregnant women (Roman chamomile in high concentrations)

- Keep away from eyes and mucous membranes
- Use only under guidance for children and infants

Interesting Facts

- Chamomile means "earth apple" in Greek, due to its apple-like scent.
- Used in traditional herbal teas for centuries as a sleep and digestive aid.
- Chamazulene, found in German chamomile, gives it its distinct blue color and strong anti-inflammatory properties.

7.10 Clove Bud Essential Oil

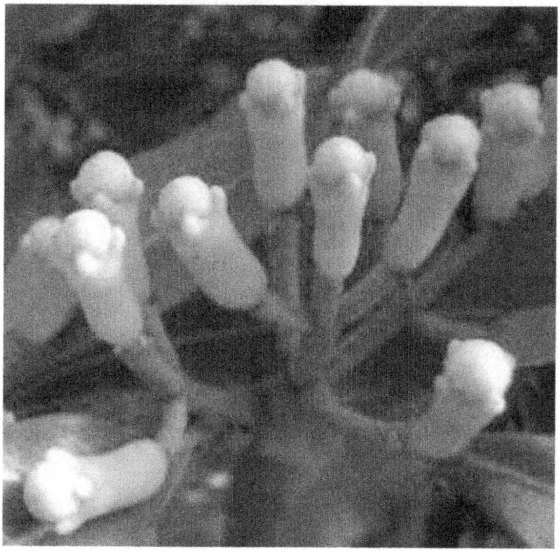

Introduction

Clove Bud Essential Oil is derived from the dried flower buds of the Syzygium aromaticum tree, native to Indonesia and cultivated in many tropical regions. Clove has been used for over 2,000 years in traditional Chinese medicine, Ayurveda, and Unani systems for its analgesic, antimicrobial, and warming properties.

The oil is rich in eugenol, which gives it powerful pain-relieving, antiseptic, and antioxidant qualities. Clove oil is commonly used in oral care, pain relief blends, and antiseptic preparations.

Botanical Information

- BOTANICAL NAME: *Syzygium aromaticum*
- FAMILY: Myrtaceae
- PLANT PART USED: Dried flower buds

- EXTRACTION METHOD: Steam Distillation
- APPEARANCE: Clear to pale yellow
- AROMA: Warm, spicy, woody, and strong

Chemical Composition (Main Constituents)

- Eugenol (up to 70–85%) – strong antiseptic & pain-reliever
- Eugenyl acetate – anti-inflammatory
- Beta-caryophyllene – soothing and calming
- Isoeugenol
- Vanillin (trace) – adds a slight sweetness

Therapeutic Properties

- Analgesic – pain-relieving
- Antiseptic – prevents infection
- Antiviral
- Antifungal
- Antibacterial
- Anti-inflammatory
- Antioxidant
- Carminative – relieves flatulence
- Insecticidal – repels insects

Benefits Of Clove Bud Essential Oil

1. Natural Pain Relief

- Highly effective for toothaches, gum pain, and sore muscles
- Commonly found in dental care products

2. Powerful Antimicrobial Agent

- Kills bacteria, fungi, and viruses
- Can be used in natural disinfectant sprays

3. Improves Oral Health

- Reduces bad breath, gum infections, and mouth ulcers
- Used in tooth powders, mouthwashes, and toothpastes

4. Supports Digestion

- Relieves bloating, indigestion, gas, and nausea
- Stimulates digestive enzymes (when used under professional supervision)

5. Anti-inflammatory for Skin & Muscles

- Eases arthritis, muscle soreness, and joint pain
- Used in massage oils and balms

6. Enhances Immunity

- Due to its antioxidant content, it helps combat oxidative stress
- Often used in immune-boosting diffuser blends

Uses Of Clove Bud Essential Oil

Aromatherapy:

- Diffused to reduce mental fatigue, purify air, and fight microbes

Topical Application (Diluted):

- Applied on gums, joints, or muscles for pain relief
- Mixed with carrier oils like coconut or olive oil

In Oral Care:

- A drop diluted in coconut oil can be used for oil pulling

Massage:

- Blended into muscle rubs for relief from soreness and stiffness

Blends Well With:

- Cinnamon
- Orange
- Lemon
- Eucalyptus
- Lavender
- Rosemary
- Tea Tree

Precautions

- Highly potent – use only in low concentrations (0.5–1%) when applying to skin
- Can cause skin irritation or sensitization if undiluted
- Not safe for infants, small children, or during pregnancy unless under medical supervision
- Do not ingest without expert guidance – can be toxic in large doses
- Avoid contact with eyes, ears, and mucous membranes

Interesting Facts

- Clove has been used in Ayurveda for centuries to enhance Agni (digestive fire).
- In ancient China, clove was chewed before speaking to the emperor – due to its breath-freshening properties.
- Eugenol in clove is used in dental anesthesia and is known to numb pain almost instantly.

7.11 Cedarwood Essential Oil

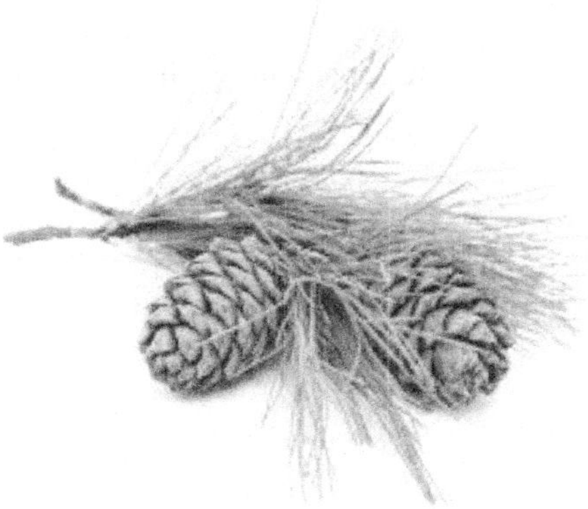

Introduction

Cedarwood essential oil is a woody, warm, and balsamic-scented oil obtained from the wood of cedar trees belonging to the *Cupressaceae* family. It has been used for centuries in aromatherapy, perfumery, and medicine for its calming, antiseptic, and insect-repelling properties.

Botanical Source

- Botanical Name: *Cedrus atlantica*, *Cedrus deodara*, *Juniperus virginiana*
- Family: *Cupressaceae*
- Common Names: Cedarwood, Himalayan Cedar, Atlas Cedar
- Part Used: Wood, sawdust, or roots
- Origin: Native to Himalayas, North America, and North Africa

Extraction Method

Cedarwood essential oil is obtained by steam distillation of wood pieces or sawdust.
The yield of essential oil is usually 2–3% depending on the species and age of the tree.

Chemical Composition

Major constituents include:

- Cedrol
- Thujopsene
- Cedrene
- Alpha-cedrene
- Widdrol

These compounds contribute to its sedative, antiseptic, and anti-inflammatory effects.

Aromatic Profile

- Scent: Woody, sweet, and balsamic
- Note: Base note in perfumery
- Blends Well With: Bergamot, Lavender, Sandalwood, Rose, Lemon, Vetiver

Therapeutic Benefits of Cedarwood Essential Oil

Category	Benefits	Mechanism / Use
1. Nervous System	Reduces stress, anxiety, and promotes calmness	Inhalation of cedrol influences limbic system to induce relaxation
2. Respiratory System	Eases cough, bronchitis, and congestion	Acts as an expectorant and anti-inflammatory agent
3. Skin Care	Useful for acne, eczema, dandruff	Antiseptic and sebum-regulating properties
4. Hair Care	Promotes hair growth, prevents hair fall	Improves scalp circulation; used in scalp massage
5. Insect Repellent	Repels moths, mosquitoes, ants	Cedrol and thujopsene act as natural insect deterrents
6. Musculoskeletal	Relieves joint pain and stiffness	Anti-inflammatory and analgesic properties
7. Emotional Wellness	Enhances grounding and focus	Commonly used in aromatherapy for meditation

Precautions

- Avoid during pregnancy.
- May cause skin irritation in sensitive individuals — perform patch test.
- Use in **diluted form** (1–2% in carrier oil).

7.12 Cypress Essential Oil

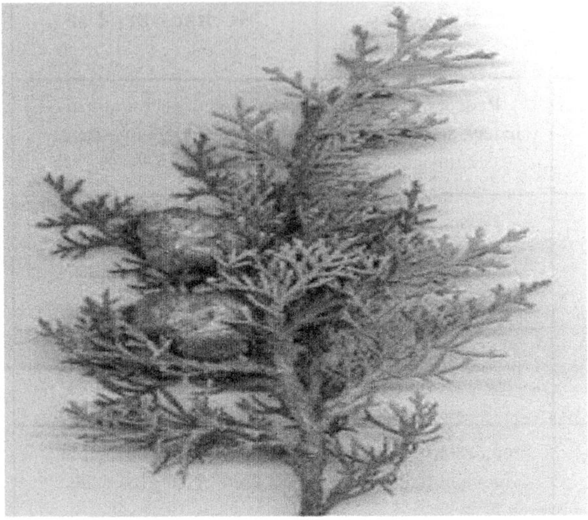

Introduction

Cypress essential oil is a refreshing, woody, and slightly spicy oil distilled from the twigs, stems, and needles of the *Cupressus sempervirens* tree. Known for its circulatory, antiseptic, and calming effects, it has been traditionally used in aromatherapy, massage, and skincare to support emotional balance and physical wellness.

Botanical Source

- Botanical Name: *Cupressus sempervirens*
- Family: *Cupressaceae*
- Common Name: Mediterranean Cypress, Italian Cypress
- Part Used: Needles, twigs, and cones
- Origin: Native to the Mediterranean region, cultivated worldwide

Extraction Method

- Method: *Steam Distillation*
- Yield: 1–2%
- Color: Pale yellow to greenish
- Aroma: Fresh, woody, balsamic

Chemical Composition

Main constituents include:

- α-pinene
- δ-3-carene
- Cedrol
- Sabinene
- Limonene

These components contribute to its astringent, antiseptic, and sedative properties.

Aromatic Profile

- Note: Middle note
- Blends Well With: Lemon, Lavender, Clary Sage, Sandalwood, Juniper Berry

Therapeutic Benefits of Cypress Essential Oil

System / Area	Therapeutic Benefits	Mechanism / Application
1. Circulatory System	Improves blood flow, reduces varicose veins, and edema	Acts as a vasoconstrictor and strengthens capillaries
2. Respiratory System	Relieves coughs, bronchitis, and congestion	Expectorant and antispasmodic effects
3. Musculoskeletal System	Eases muscle cramps, rheumatism, and fatigue	Enhances circulation and reduces lactic acid build-up
4. Nervous System	promotes calmness, relieves emotional stress	Has mild sedative and grounding effects
5. Skin Care	Tightens skin, reduces excessive sweating, helps oily skin	Astringent and toning properties
6. Menstrual / Reproductive	Helps regulate menstrual cycle, eases PMS cramps	Hormone-balancing and antispasmodic actions
7. Detoxification	Supports lymphatic drainage	Stimulates the lymphatic system to clear toxins

Precautions

- Avoid use during pregnancy.
- For external use only — always dilute in a carrier oil.
- Conduct a patch test before applying to skin.

7.13 Clary Sage Essential Oil

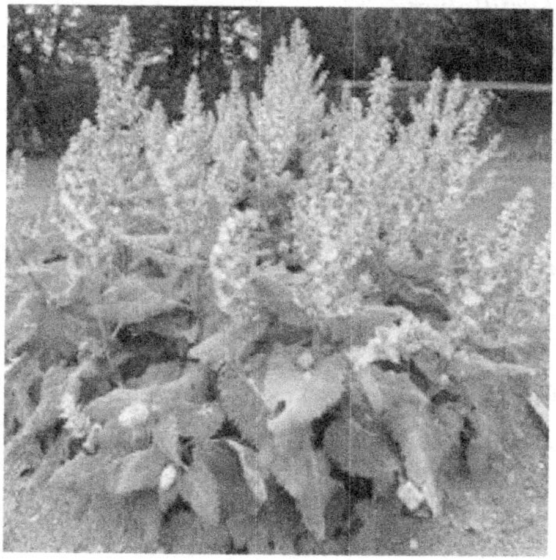

Introduction

Clary Sage essential oil is a sweet, herbaceous, and floral-scented oil obtained from the flowering tops and leaves of *Salvia sclarea*. It is highly valued in aromatherapy and natural medicine for its calming, hormone-balancing, and antidepressant properties. Traditionally, it has been used to support women's health, stress relief, and skin care.

Botanical Source

- Botanical Name: *Salvia sclarea*
- Family: *Lamiaceae*
- Common Name: Clary Sage
- Part Used: Flowering tops and leaves
- Origin: Native to Southern Europe and Mediterranean region

Extraction Method

- Method: *Steam Distillation*
- Part Used: Flowering tops and leaves
- Yield: 0.2–0.4%
- Color: Pale yellow to golden
- Aroma: Sweet, nutty, herbaceous, slightly floral

Chemical Composition

Main constituents:

- Linalyl acetate (45–75%)
- Linalool
- Germacrene D
- Sclareol
- Caryophyllene

These active compounds contribute to the antidepressant, sedative, and hormone-regulating properties of clary sage oil.

Aromatic Profile

- Note: Middle to top note
- Blends Well With: Lavender, Geranium, Bergamot, Sandalwood, Lemon, Patchouli

Therapeutic Benefits of Clary Sage Essential Oil

System / Area	Therapeutic Benefits	Mechanism / Application
1. Nervous System	Reduces stress, anxiety, and depression	Acts as a natural sedative and balances serotonin levels
2. Hormonal System	Balances estrogen levels, helps with PMS and menopause	Sclareol mimics estrogen activity

3. Reproductive System	Eases menstrual cramps and supports uterine health	Antispasmodic and hormone-regulating
4. Skin Care	Improves oily skin, tones, and reduces inflammation	Astringent and antibacterial properties
5. Hair Care	Strengthens hair, reduces dandruff	Regulates scalp sebum
6. Musculoskeletal System	Relieves muscle spasms and fatigue	Antispasmodic and anti-inflammatory
7. Emotional Wellness	Promotes relaxation, confidence, and clarity	Used in aromatherapy and meditation practices

Precautions

- Avoid using oil during pregnancy (especially early months).
- May cause drowsiness — avoid driving immediately after use.
- Use in diluted form for topical application (1–2%).
- Avoid alcohol consumption soon after inhalation or massage

7.14 Eucalyptus Essential Oil

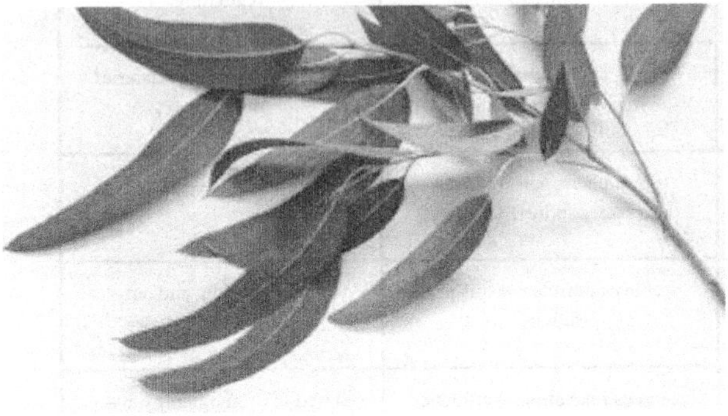

Introduction

Eucalyptus essential oil is one of the most widely used therapeutic oils, known for its fresh, camphoraceous aroma and strong antiseptic, antiviral, and expectorant properties. It is extracted from the leaves of Eucalyptus trees, native to Australia. Traditionally, it has been used for respiratory ailments, wound healing, and pain relief.

Botanical Source

- Botanical Name: *Eucalyptus globulus*
- Family: *Myrtaceae*
- Common Name: Blue Gum Tree
- Part Used: Fresh or partially dried leaves and young twigs
- Origin: Australia, India, China, Spain

Extraction Method

- Method: *Steam Distillation*
- Part Used: Fresh leaves and twigs

- Yield: 1–3%
- Color: Colorless to pale yellow
- Aroma: Fresh, sharp, and camphor-like

Chemical Composition

Major constituents include:

- 1,8-Cineole (Eucalyptol) – 70–85%
- α-Pinene
- Limonene
- Globulol
- Terpineol

These components contribute to its antimicrobial, expectorant, analgesic, and anti-inflammatory actions.

Aromatic Profile

- Note: Top note
- Blends Well With: Lemon, Peppermint, Lavender, Rosemary, Tea Tree

Therapeutic Benefits of Eucalyptus Essential Oil

System / Area	Therapeutic Benefits	Mechanism / Application
1. Respiratory System	Relieves cough, asthma, sinusitis, bronchitis	Acts as expectorant; clears nasal and bronchial congestion
2. Nervous System	Refreshes mind, relieves fatigue and headaches	Stimulates mental clarity through inhalation
3. Musculoskeletal System	Eases joint pain, muscle aches, arthritis	Anti-inflammatory and analgesic properties
4. Immune System	Boosts immunity, fights infections	Antiviral and antibacterial effects
5. Skin Care	Helps heal wounds, insect bites, and acne	Antiseptic and cooling properties
6. Oral Health	Prevents bad breath, gum infections	Antibacterial and anti-inflammatory actions
7. Environment / Hygiene	Acts as natural disinfectant and insect repellent	Used in vaporizers, diffusers, and cleaning sprays

Precautions

- Avoid use in **infants or small children** (due to high cineole content).
- Use **diluted** on skin (1–2%).
- Avoid contact with eyes and mucous membranes.
- Do not ingest without professional guidance.

7.15 Fennel Essential Oil

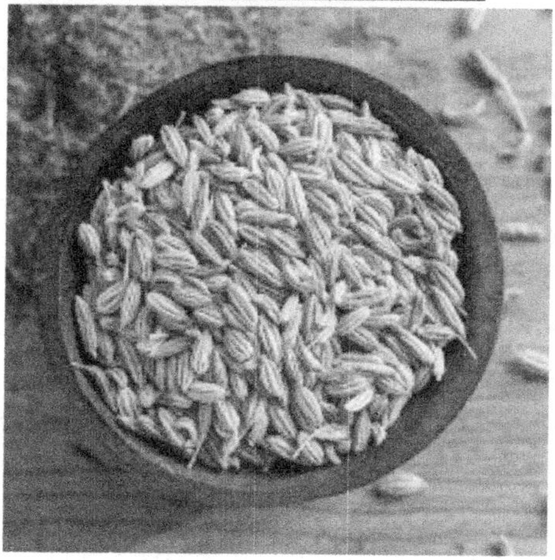

Introduction

Fennel essential oil is a sweet, spicy, and anise-like aromatic oil extracted from the crushed seeds of the fennel plant (*Foeniculum vulgare*). It is known for its digestive, detoxifying, and hormone-balancing properties. Used since ancient times by the Greeks and Egyptians, fennel oil remains a popular choice in aromatherapy and herbal medicine for improving digestion, regulating hormones, and detoxifying the body.

Botanical Source

- Botanical Name: *Foeniculum vulgare*
- Family: *Apiaceae* (Umbelliferae)
- Common Name: Fennel
- Part Used: Crushed seeds
- Origin: Native to the Mediterranean region; cultivated in India, China, and Europe

Extraction Method

- Method: *Steam Distillation*
- Part Used: Seeds (dried and crushed)
- Yield: 2–6%
- Color: Clear to pale yellow
- Aroma: Sweet, spicy, licorice-like

Chemical Composition

Major constituents include:

- Anethole (50–70%)
- Fenchone (5–20%)
- Estragole (methyl chavicol)
- Limonene
- α-pinene

These compounds are responsible for fennel oil's carminative, antispasmodic, estrogenic, and detoxifying effects.

Aromatic Profile

- Note: Middle note
- Blends Well With: Geranium, Lavender, Lemon, Sandalwood, Rose, and Bergamot

Therapeutic Benefits of Fennel Essential Oil

System / Area	Therapeutic Benefits	Mechanism / Application
1. Digestive System	Relieves indigestion, bloating, gas, and constipation	Stimulates peristalsis and digestive secretions
2. Endocrine & Hormonal System	Balances hormones, supports menstrual cycle, eases menopause	Contains phytoestrogen-like compound anethole
3. Respiratory System	Clears mucus, eases cough and bronchitis	Acts as an expectorant
4. Detoxification	Promotes liver health and eliminates toxins	Stimulates metabolic function
5. Nervous System	Reduces mental fatigue and promotes clarity	Has mild stimulant and mood-lifting properties
6. Skin Care	Tones skin and reduces puffiness	Antioxidant and detoxifying effects
7. Musculoskeletal System	Eases cramps and muscular spasms	Antispasmodic action on smooth muscles

Precautions

- Avoid use during pregnancy and breastfeeding.
- Not suitable for epileptic patients (contains fenchone).
- Use diluted on skin (1–2%) to prevent irritation.
- Avoid internal use without professional guidance.

7.16 Frankincense Essential Oil

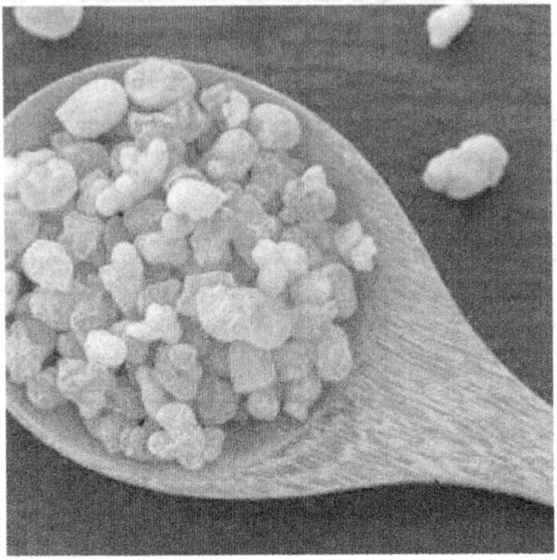

Introduction

Frankincense essential oil—often called the "King of Oils"—is a sweet, woody, balsamic, and slightly spicy aromatic oil obtained from the resin of *Boswellia* trees. It has been treasured for centuries in spiritual rituals, medicine, and perfumery. Traditionally used in Ayurvedic, Egyptian, and biblical healing, frankincense supports respiratory health, skin regeneration, emotional balance, and immunity.

Botanical Source

- Botanical Name: *Boswellia carterii*, *Boswellia serrata*, or *Boswellia sacra*
- Family: *Burseraceae*
- Common Name: Olibanum or Indian Frankincense
- Part Used: Gum resin (oleo-gum-resin) exuded from bark incisions
- Origin: Native to Arabia, Somalia, India, and Northeast Africa

Extraction Method

- Method: *Steam Distillation* of the resin (gum)
- Yield: 3–10%
- Color: Pale yellow to amber
- Aroma: Warm, sweet, woody, balsamic

Chemical Composition

Major constituents include:

- α-Pinene (30–50%)
- Limonene
- Incensole acetate
- β-Caryophyllene
- Octyl acetate
- Terpinen-4-ol

These compounds are responsible for frankincense's anti-inflammatory, antiseptic, sedative, and rejuvenating effects.

Aromatic Profile

- Note: Base note
- Blends Well With: Myrrh, Sandalwood, Bergamot, Lavender, Geranium, Lemon

Therapeutic Benefits of Frankincense Essential Oil

System / Area	Therapeutic Benefits	Mechanism / Application
1. Respiratory System	Relieves cough, asthma, and congestion	Acts as expectorant and anti-inflammatory
2. Nervous System	Reduces anxiety, depression, and stress	Sedative effects on limbic system; promotes calmness
3. Skin Care	Reduces scars, wrinkles, acne, and wounds	Stimulates cell regeneration and has astringent action
4. Immune System	Strengthens immunity, combats infections	Boosts white blood cell activity
5. Musculoskeletal System	Eases arthritis, muscle pain, and inflammation	Boswellic acids act as anti-inflammatory agents
6. Spiritual / Emotional	Enhances meditation, grounding, and focus	Traditionally used for spiritual clarity
7. Digestive System	Aids digestion, reduces bloating	Promotes secretion of digestive enzymes

Precautions

- Non-toxic and non-irritant in general use.
- Use diluted for topical applications (1–2%).
- Avoid internal use without medical supervision.
- Store away from direct sun

7.17 Geranium Essential Oil

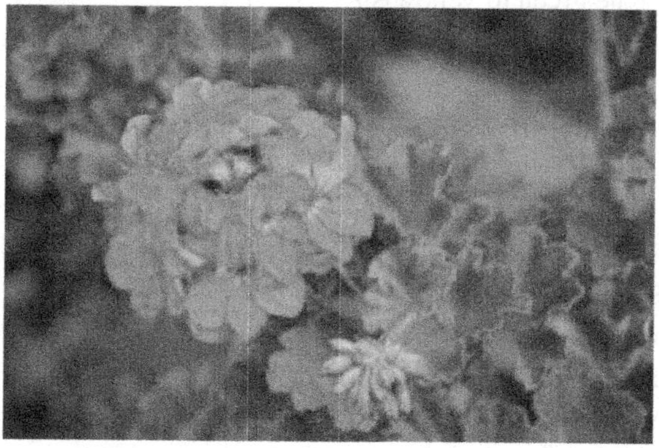

Introduction

Geranium essential oil is a sweet, floral, and rosy-scented oil extracted from the leaves and stems of the *Pelargonium graveolens* plant. It is highly valued in aromatherapy for its balancing, uplifting, and skin-regenerating effects. Traditionally, it has been used to promote emotional stability, hormonal balance, and skin health.

Botanical Source

- Botanical Name: *Pelargonium graveolens*
- Family: *Geraniaceae*
- Common Name: Rose Geranium, Sweet Geranium
- Part Used: Leaves, stems, and flowers
- Origin: Native to South Africa; cultivated in Egypt, India, China, and France

Extraction Method

- Method: *Steam Distillation*
- Part Used: Fresh leaves and stems

- Yield: 0.1–0.3%
- Color: Pale green to yellowish
- Aroma: Sweet, floral, rosy, herbaceous

Chemical Composition

Main constituents include:

- Citronellol
- Geraniol
- Linalool
- Citronellyl formate
- Menthone
- Isomenthone

These compounds contribute to its antimicrobial, anti-inflammatory, balancing, and skin-toning properties.

Aromatic Profile

- Note: Middle note
- Blends Well With: Lavender, Rose, Bergamot, Clary Sage, Sandalwood, Lemon

Therapeutic Benefits of Geranium Essential Oil

System / Area	Therapeutic Benefits	Mechanism / Application
1. Skin Care	Improves complexion, reduces acne, eczema, and scars	Regulates sebum and promotes skin regeneration
2. Hormonal System	Balances hormones, relieves PMS and menopause symptoms	Acts as an adaptogen on endocrine glands
3. Nervous System	Reduces stress, anxiety, and depression	Calming and uplifting aroma affects limbic system
4. Circulatory System	Improves blood flow, reduces varicose veins and swelling	Vasoconstrictive and tonic properties
5. Immune System	Boosts immunity and fights infections	Antibacterial and antifungal properties
6. Musculoskeletal System	Relieves muscle cramps and fatigue	Mild anti-inflammatory and relaxing effect
7. Wound Healing	Promotes clotting and speeds up healing	Astringent and antimicrobial actions

Precautions

- Generally non-toxic and non-irritant.
- Should be diluted before topical application.
- Avoid use during early pregnancy (as a precaution).
- Store in a cool, dark place away from sunlight.

7.18 Ginger Essential Oil

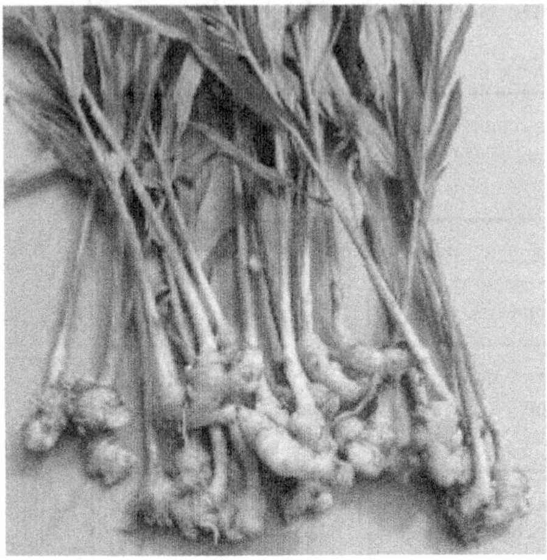

Introduction

Ginger essential oil is a warm, spicy, and energizing oil extracted from the rhizomes of *Zingiber officinale*. Known for its digestive, anti-inflammatory, and circulatory-stimulating effects, it has been used for centuries in Ayurveda and traditional Chinese medicine. It is often called the "oil of empowerment" for its ability to uplift mood and strengthen vitality.

Botanical Source

- Botanical Name: *Zingiber officinale*
- Family: *Zingiberaceae*
- Common Name: Ginger
- Part Used: Rhizome (root)
- Origin: Native to India and Southeast Asia

Extraction Method

- Method: *Steam Distillation*
- Part Used: Dried or fresh rhizomes
- Yield: 1–3%
- Color: Pale yellow to amber
- Aroma: Warm, spicy, woody, and earthy

Chemical Composition

Main constituents include:

- Zingiberene (20–30%)
- β-Sesquiphellandrene
- α-Farnesene
- Camphene
- Citral
- Gingerol and Shogaol (trace amounts)

These compounds give the oil its antioxidant, anti-inflammatory, digestive, and warming properties.

Aromatic Profile

- **Note:** Middle to base note
- **Blends Well With:** Lemon, Orange, Clove, Cinnamon, Rosemary, Eucalyptus, Sandalwood

Therapeutic Benefits of Ginger Essential Oil

System / Area	Therapeutic Benefits	Mechanism / Application
1. Digestive System	Relieves nausea, vomiting, gas, and indigestion	Stimulates digestive enzymes and peristalsis
2. Musculoskeletal System	Reduces joint pain, arthritis, and muscle stiffness	Anti-inflammatory and warming analgesic effect
3. Circulatory System	Improves blood circulation and warms the body	Vasodilator action; enhances oxygen flow
4. Respiratory System	Eases cold, cough, and flu symptoms	Acts as an expectorant and antimicrobial
5. Nervous System	Boosts energy, confidence, and motivation	Stimulating and grounding aroma
6. Immune System	Strengthens immunity and fights infections	Antioxidant and antimicrobial activity
7. Skin & Hair	Improves skin tone and reduces dandruff	Increases circulation and detoxification

Precautions

- Use diluted (1–2%) for topical applications to avoid skin irritation.
- Avoid use during pregnancy without medical advice.
- Avoid contact with eyes and mucous membranes.
- Internal use only under expert supervision.

7.19 Juniper Berry Essential Oil

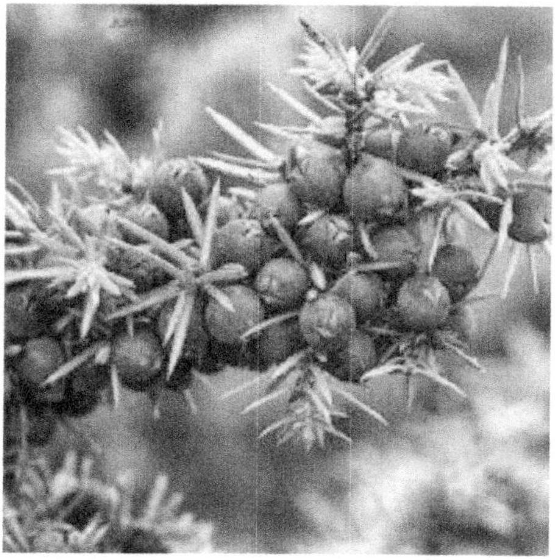

Introduction

Juniper berry essential oil is a fresh, woody, and slightly sweet oil derived from the berries of the *Juniperus communis* tree. It is widely used in aromatherapy and herbal medicine for its detoxifying, purifying, and calming properties. Traditionally, it has been employed to cleanse the body, boost kidney function, and relieve muscle tension.

Botanical Source

- Botanical Name: *Juniperus communis*
- Family: *Cupressaceae*
- Common Name: Juniper, Common Juniper
- Part Used: Berries (sometimes needles)
- Origin: Native to Europe, North America, and parts of Asia

Extraction Method

- Method: *Steam Distillation*
- Part Used: Dried ripe berries
- Yield: 1–2%
- Color: Colorless to pale yellow
- Aroma: Fresh, woody, balsamic, crisp

Chemical Composition

Main constituents include:

- α-Pinene (20–50%)
- Myrcene
- Sabinene
- Limonene
- β-Pinene
- Cadinene
- Bornyl acetate

These components contribute to the oil's antiseptic, diuretic, detoxifying, and soothing properties.

Aromatic Profile

- Note: Middle note
- Blends Well With: Cypress, Cedarwood, Rosemary, Lavender, Lemon, Sandalwood

Therapeutic Benefits of Juniper Berry Essential Oil

System / Area	Therapeutic Benefits	Mechanism / Application
1. Detoxification	Helps eliminate toxins and reduces fluid retention	Stimulates kidney and lymphatic system
2. Skin Care	Treats acne, oily skin, and eczema	Astringent and antibacterial effects
3. Musculoskeletal System	Relieves muscle aches, arthritis, and joint pain	Anti-inflammatory and warming properties
4. Nervous System	Reduces anxiety, stress, and mental fatigue	Calming and grounding aroma
5. Immune System	Boosts immunity and protects from infections	Antiseptic and antioxidant properties
6. Digestive System	Relieves bloating, gas, and indigestion	Stimulates digestion and reduces spasms
7. Urinary System	Acts as a natural diuretic	Promotes urine flow and helps prevent infections

Precautions

- Avoid use during pregnancy and in cases of kidney disorders.
- Always dilute before topical application.
- Avoid prolonged use — use intermittently.
- Perform a patch test before applying on skin.

7.20 Lavender Essential Oil

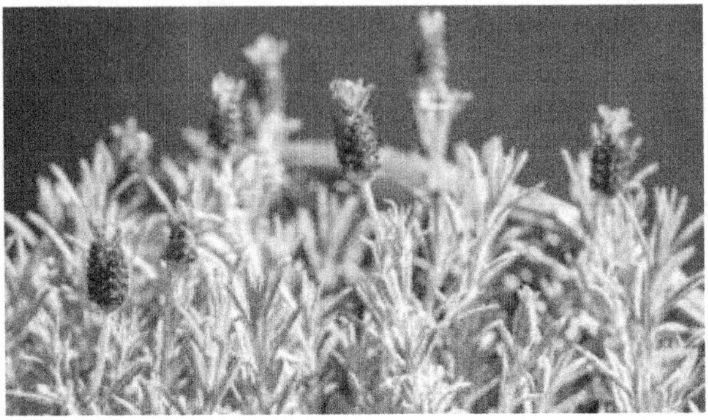

Introduction

Lavender essential oil is one of the most popular and versatile essential oils in aromatherapy. Extracted from the flowers of *Lavandula angustifolia*, it is valued for its calming, relaxing, antiseptic, and healing properties. It is widely used to promote sleep, relieve stress, soothe skin irritations, and support emotional well-being.

Botanical Source

- **Botanical Name:** *Lavandula angustifolia* (syn. *Lavandula officinalis*)
- **Family:** *Lamiaceae*
- **Common Name:** True Lavender, English Lavender
- **Part Used:** Flowers and flowering tops
- **Origin:** Native to the Mediterranean region; cultivated globally in France, India, Bulgaria, and England

Extraction Method

- Method: *Steam Distillation*
- Part Used: Fresh flowering tops
- Yield: 1–3%

- Color: Colorless to pale yellow
- Aroma: Floral, sweet, herbaceous, and refreshing

Chemical Composition

Main constituents include:

- Linalool (20–45%)
- Linalyl acetate (25–46%)
- Lavandulol
- 1,8-Cineole
- Camphor
- Geraniol

These compounds give lavender its calming, antiseptic, anti-inflammatory, and sedative actions.

Aromatic Profile

- Note: Top to middle note
- Blends Well With: Bergamot, Lemon, Rose, Cedarwood, Clary Sage, Geranium, and Rosemary

Therapeutic Benefits of Lavender Essential Oil

System / Area	Therapeutic Benefits	Mechanism / Application
1. Nervous System	Reduces stress, anxiety, and depression	Calming effect on the nervous system; regulates cortisol levels
2. Sleep & Relaxation	Promotes restful sleep and eases insomnia	Sedative aroma enhances GABA activity in the brain
3. Skin Care	Heals acne, burns, insect bites, and eczema	Antiseptic, anti-inflammatory, and regenerative properties
4. Musculoskeletal System	Relieves pain, cramps, and muscle tension	Improves blood circulation and reduces inflammation
5. Respiratory System	Eases cold, flu, and sinus congestion	Mucolytic and antimicrobial activity
6. Circulatory System	Lowers blood pressure and enhances blood flow	Relaxing and vasodilatory properties
7. Emotional Health	Balances mood, promotes clarity, and relieves fatigue	Soothing aroma harmonizes mind and body

Precautions

- Generally non-toxic and non-irritant when diluted.
- Avoid contact with eyes and mucous membranes.
- Safe for children and elderly in small doses.
- Pregnant women should use under medical advice.

7.21 Lemon Essential Oil

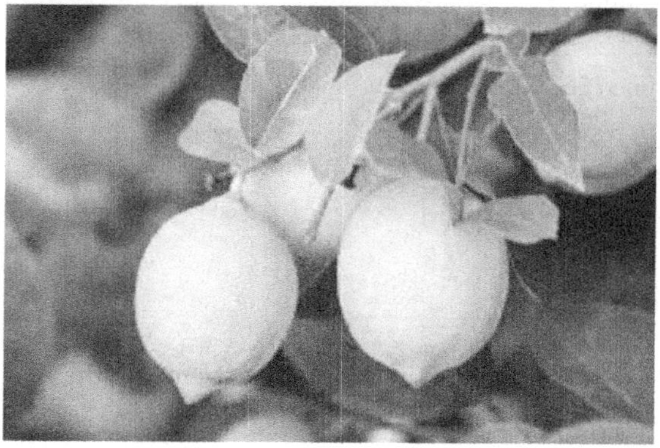

Introduction

Lemon essential oil is a fresh, bright, and citrusy oil extracted from the peel of the lemon fruit (*Citrus limon*). Widely used in aromatherapy, skincare, and household cleaning, it is valued for its energizing, uplifting, antimicrobial, and detoxifying properties.

Botanical Source

- Botanical Name: *Citrus limon*
- Family: *Rutaceae*
- Common Name: Lemon
- Part Used: Fresh peel (zest)
- Origin: Native to Asia; cultivated globally in Mediterranean countries, USA, and India

Extraction Method

- **Method:** *Cold Pressed (Expression) of Peel*
- **Yield:** 0.5–3%
- **Color:** Pale yellow
- **Aroma:** Fresh, citrusy, bright, and sweet

Chemical Composition

Main constituents include:

- Limonene (50–70%)
- β-Pinene
- γ-Terpinene
- Citral
- Neral
- Geranial

These compounds give lemon oil its antioxidant, antimicrobial, detoxifying, and uplifting properties.

Aromatic Profile

- **Note:** Top note
- **Blends Well With:** Lavender, Rosemary, Peppermint, Frankincense, Eucalyptus, Bergamot

Therapeutic Benefits of Lemon Essential Oil

System / Area	Therapeutic Benefits	Mechanism / Application
1. Immune System	Strengthens immunity, fights infections	Antimicrobial and antiviral activity
2. Skin Care	Brightens skin, reduces acne, detoxifies	Antioxidant, astringent, and cleansing properties
3. Digestive System	Aids digestion, relieves bloating, nausea	Stimulates digestive secretions and detoxification
4. Nervous System	Reduces mental fatigue, stress, and anxiety	Uplifting and energizing aroma stimulates mood
5. Respiratory System	Clears nasal congestion and supports lungs	Expectorant and antimicrobial effects
6. Detoxification	Promotes liver function and lymphatic drainage	Stimulates elimination of toxins
7. Household Uses	Natural disinfectant and deodorizer	Cleans surfaces and purifies air

Precautions

- Avoid direct sun exposure after topical application (phototoxic).
- Always dilute before skin use (1–2%).
- Avoid in infants and sensitive skin.
- Store in dark glass bottles away from heat and light.

7.22 Lemongrass Essential Oil

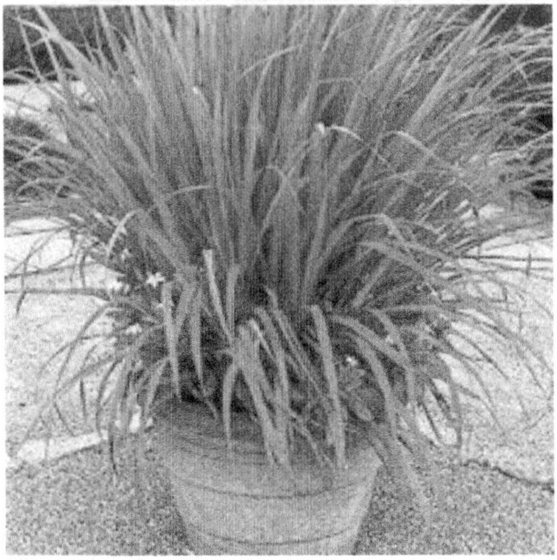

Introduction

Lemongrass essential oil is a highly aromatic oil extracted from the leaves and stalks of the lemongrass plant (*Cymbopogon spp.*), a tropical grass native to India, Sri Lanka, and Southeast Asia. Known for its fresh, citrusy scent, lemongrass oil has been widely used in traditional medicine, aromatherapy, and cosmetics for centuries.

This oil is especially valued for its antibacterial, antifungal, anti-inflammatory, and analgesic properties. It plays a significant role in natural healing systems like Ayurveda and Traditional Chinese Medicine, where it is used to treat fevers, infections, digestive issues, and muscle pain.

Botanical Information

- Botanical Name: *Cymbopogon citratus* (West Indian) / *Cymbopogon flexuosus* (East Indian)
- Family: Poaceae (grass family)

- Part Used: Leaves and stalks
- Extraction Method: Steam distillation
- Color: Pale yellow to deep yellow
- Aroma: Fresh, lemony, earthy, slightly bitter

Major Chemical Constituents

Compound	Function
Citral (Neral & Geranial)	Strong antimicrobial, anti-inflammatory, citrus scent
Geraniol	Antioxidant, antifungal
Myrcene	Analgesic, anti-inflammatory
Limonene	Cleansing, uplifting, antibacterial
Linalool	Relaxant, sedative, skin-soothing

Note: The exact composition can vary depending on the region and species.

Therapeutic Properties

- Antimicrobial (antibacterial, antifungal, antiviral)
- Anti-inflammatory
- Antioxidant
- Analgesic (pain relief)
- Astringent
- Insecticidal
- Sedative (mild)
- Digestive stimulant

Aromatherapy & Emotional Use

- Uplifting and energizing: Boosts mood and reduces mental fatigue
- Reduces anxiety and depression: Often used in stress-relief blends
- Promotes mental clarity: Improves focus and alertness

Popular Diffuser Blend Example:

- 3 drops Lemongrass
- 2 drops Lavender
- 2 drops Eucalyptus

Topical Applications

Always dilute in a carrier oil (e.g., coconut oil, sweet almond oil)

- For muscle pain or joint stiffness: Massage into sore areas
- For acne and oily skin: Used in diluted form in facial toners
- As an insect repellent: Effective against mosquitoes and houseflies

Household & Practical Uses

- Air freshener and deodorizer: Kills odor-causing bacteria
- Natural insect repellent: Common in sprays and candles
- Surface cleaner: Mixed with vinegar and water for cleaning

Safety and Precautions

- Skin Sensitivity: Can cause irritation if undiluted
- Phototoxicity: Not phototoxic, but still patch-test first
- Pregnancy/Nursing: Avoid in high concentrations

- Children: Not recommended for children under 2
- Pets: Use cautiously around cats and dogs

Storage

- Store in a cool, dark place
- Keep tightly sealed to prevent oxidation
- Shelf life: 2–3 years if stored properly

7.23 Marjoram Essential Oil

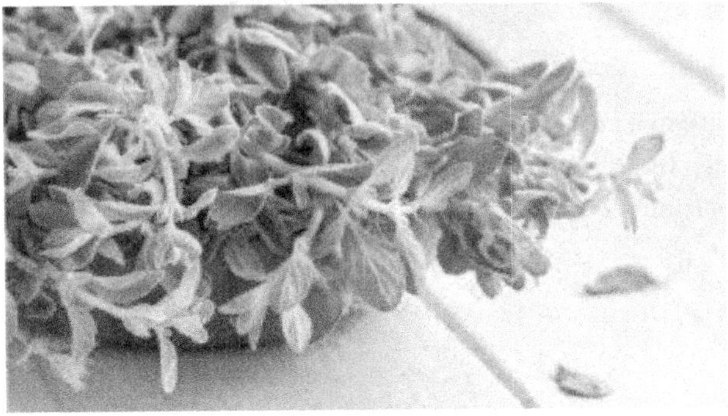

Introduction

Marjoram essential oil, derived from the leaves and flowering tops of *Origanum majorana*, is a warm, sweet, herbaceous oil renowned for its calming, analgesic, and digestive properties. Often called "herbal pain relief oil", it has been traditionally used in aromatherapy, herbal medicine, and massage therapy for relaxing muscles, improving sleep, and supporting respiratory and circulatory health.

Botanical Source

- Botanical Name: *Origanum majorana*
- Family: *Lamiaceae*
- Common Name: Sweet Marjoram
- Part Used: Leaves and flowering tops
- Origin: Native to Mediterranean regions; cultivated in Egypt, Morocco, and India

Extraction Method

- Method: *Steam Distillation*
- Part Used: Fresh or partially dried leaves and flowering tops

- Yield: 0.2–0.5%
- Color: Pale yellow to amber
- Aroma: Sweet, warm, herbaceous, slightly woody

Chemical Composition

Main constituents include:

- Terpinen-4-ol
- Sabinene hydrate
- α-Terpinene
- Linalool
- γ-Terpinene
- Cineole (small amount)

These compounds are responsible for its antispasmodic, analgesic, antimicrobial, and calming effects.

Aromatic Profile

- Note: Middle note
- Blends Well With: Lavender, Bergamot, Rosemary, Thyme, Clary Sage, Lemon

Therapeutic Benefits of Marjoram Essential Oil

System / Area	Therapeutic Benefits	Mechanism / Application
1. Nervous System	Reduces anxiety, stress, and promotes sleep	Sedative and calming effect on CNS
2. Musculoskeletal System	Relieves muscle spasms, cramps, and joint pain	Antispasmodic and analgesic properties
3. Circulatory System	Improves blood circulation and reduces blood pressure	Vasodilatory and tonic effect
4. Respiratory System	Eases cough, bronchitis, and congestion	Expectorant and mild antimicrobial action
5. Digestive System	Relieves bloating, indigestion, and gas	Stimulates digestive enzymes and relaxes GI muscles
6. Immune System	Supports immunity and fights infections	Antimicrobial and antioxidant effects
7. Skin Care	Soothes minor skin irritations and promotes healing	Anti-inflammatory and antiseptic properties

Precautions

- Avoid during pregnancy and in cases of hypotension.
- Use diluted for topical applications (1–2%).
- May cause mild skin irritation in sensitive individuals.

7.24 Neroli Essential Oil

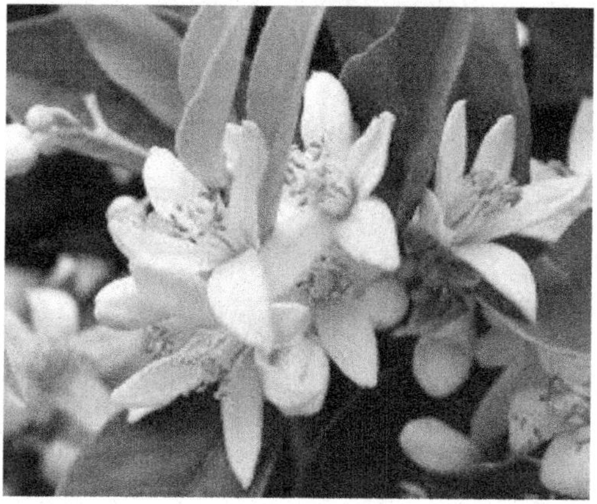

Introduction

Neroli essential oil is a sweet, floral, and citrusy oil extracted from the bitter orange blossom (*Citrus aurantium var. amara*). It is highly valued in aromatherapy and perfumery for its calming, uplifting, and skin-regenerating properties. Traditionally, neroli oil has been used for stress relief, emotional balance, and rejuvenation of the skin.

Botanical Source

- Botanical Name: *Citrus aurantium var. amara*
- Family: *Rutaceae*
- Common Name: Bitter Orange, Orange Blossom
- Part Used: Fresh flowers
- Origin: Native to Southeast Asia; cultivated in Morocco, Tunisia, Italy, and Egypt

Extraction Method

- Method: *Steam Distillation* of fresh flowers
- Yield: 0.2–0.4%
- Color: Pale yellow to amber
- Aroma: Sweet, floral, citrusy, slightly spicy

Chemical Composition

Major constituents include:

- Linalool
- Linalyl acetate
- Nerolidol
- Geraniol
- Farnesol
- Citral (trace amounts)

These compounds are responsible for neroli's antidepressant, calming, antibacterial, and skin-rejuvenating properties.

Aromatic Profile

- Note: Middle to top note
- Blends Well With: Bergamot, Lavender, Rose, Jasmine, Patchouli, Sandalwood

Therapeutic Benefits of Neroli Essential Oil

System / Area	Therapeutic Benefits	Mechanism / Application
1. Nervous System	Reduces anxiety, stress, and mild depression	Calming effect on CNS; balances mood
2. Sleep & Relaxation	Improves sleep quality and relieves insomnia	Sedative effect via olfactory stimulation
3. Skin Care	Heals scars, regenerates skin, reduces wrinkles	Antimicrobial, antioxidant, and regenerative properties
4. Circulatory System	Improves blood circulation	Promotes blood flow and relieves tension
5. Digestive System	Reduces stomach cramps and indigestion	Antispasmodic effect on smooth muscles
6. Hormonal Balance	Supports hormonal regulation and relieves PMS	Phytoestrogenic and balancing effects
7. Emotional & Spiritual	Uplifts mood, enhances meditation, emotional clarity	Used in aromatherapy and stress relief

Precautions

- Generally non-toxic and non-irritant.
- Safe for most adults and children, but should always be diluted for topical use.
- Avoid direct sunlight immediately after topical application.
- Store in dark glass bottles away from heat and light.

7.25 Orange Essential Oil

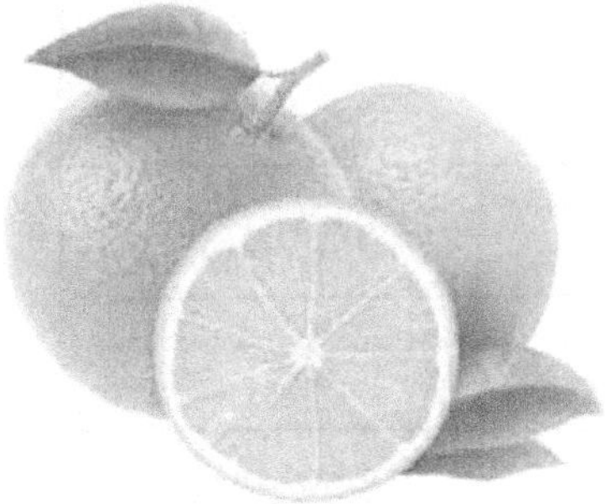

Introduction

Orange essential oil is a fresh, sweet, and citrusy oil extracted from the peel of the sweet orange fruit (*Citrus sinensis*). It is widely used in aromatherapy, perfumery, and natural cleaning products for its uplifting, calming, and antimicrobial properties. Orange oil is known to reduce stress, enhance mood, and support digestion.

Botanical Source

- Botanical Name: *Citrus sinensis*
- Family: *Rutaceae*
- Common Name: Sweet Orange
- Part Used: Fresh peel (zest)
- Origin: Native to Southeast Asia; cultivated globally in the USA, Brazil, Spain, and India

Extraction Method

- Method: *Cold Pressed / Expression of Peel*
- Yield: 0.5–3%
- Color: Pale yellow to orange
- Aroma: Sweet, fresh, citrusy, and bright

Chemical Composition

Main constituents include:

- Limonene (80–95%)
- Myrcene
- α-Pinene
- Linalool
- Citral (trace amounts)

These compounds give orange essential oil its antioxidant, antimicrobial, uplifting, and digestive properties.

Aromatic Profile

- Note: Top note
- Blends Well With: Lavender, Peppermint, Bergamot, Lemon, Geranium, Frankincense

Therapeutic Benefits of Orange Essential Oil

System / Area	Therapeutic Benefits	Mechanism / Application
1. Nervous System	Reduces anxiety, stress, and fatigue	Uplifting aroma stimulates mood and serotonin release
2. Digestive System	Improves appetite, relieves bloating, and indigestion	Stimulates digestive secretions and smooth muscle relaxation
3. Immune System	Supports immunity and fights infections	Antimicrobial and antioxidant effects
4. Skin Care	Brightens complexion, reduces oily skin	Astringent and antiseptic properties
5. Respiratory System	Clears nasal congestion and improves breathing	Mild expectorant and antimicrobial activity
6. Emotional Health	Uplifts mood, promotes positivity	Aromatherapy for stress relief and emotional balance
7. Household Uses	Natural disinfectant and deodorizer	Cleans surfaces, purifies air, and repels insects

Precautions

- Avoid direct sunlight after topical application (phototoxic).
- Dilute before skin use (1–2%).
- Avoid in infants and sensitive skin.
- Store in dark glass bottles away from heat and light.

7.26 Palmarosa Essential Oil

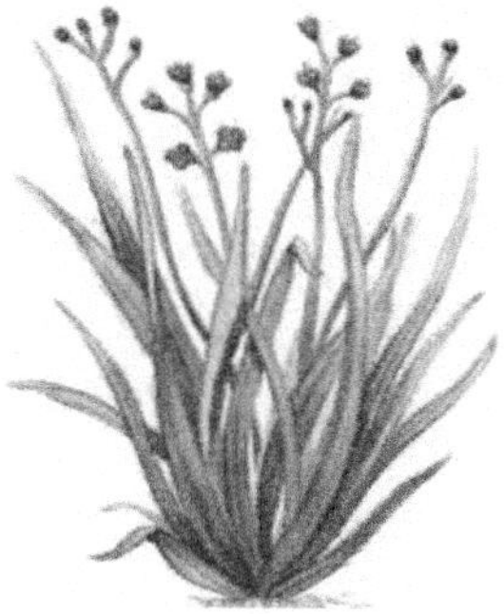

Introduction

Palmarosa essential oil is a sweet, floral, and slightly rosy oil extracted from the leaves and stems of *Cymbopogon martinii*. It is highly valued in aromatherapy, skincare, and natural medicine for its moisturizing, antibacterial, and stress-relieving properties. Palmarosa is often called the "regenerative oil" because of its skin-rejuvenating and balancing effects.

Botanical Source

- Botanical Name: *Cymbopogon martinii*
- Family: *Poaceae* (Grass family)
- Common Name: Palmarosa, Indian Geranium Grass
- Part Used: Leaves and stems
- Origin: Native to India; cultivated in Nepal, Madagascar, and Java

Extraction Method

- Method: *Steam Distillation*
- Part Used: Fresh or dried leaves and stems
- Yield: 0.5–1%
- Color: Pale yellow
- Aroma: Sweet, floral, rosy, slightly grassy

Chemical Composition

Main constituents include:

- Geraniol (70–85%)
- Myrcene
- Linalool
- Geranyl acetate
- Citronellol

These compounds give Palmarosa oil its antibacterial, antifungal, hydrating, and calming properties.

Aromatic Profile

- Note: Middle note
- Blends Well With: Lavender, Geranium, Rose, Bergamot, Lemon, Sandalwood

Therapeutic Benefits of Palmarosa Essential Oil

System / Area	Therapeutic Benefits	Mechanism / Application
1. Skin Care	Moisturizes dry skin, reduces scars, wrinkles, and acne	Regulates sebum, promotes cell regeneration
2. Nervous System	Reduces stress, anxiety, and fatigue	Calming and balancing aroma stimulates relaxation
3. Immune System	Fights bacterial and fungal infections	Antimicrobial and antifungal properties
4. Digestive System	Improves digestion and relieves bloating	Stimulates digestive secretions and smooth muscle relaxation
5. Circulatory System	Improves blood flow, reduces water retention	Vasodilatory and detoxifying effect
6. Emotional Health	Enhances mood, emotional clarity, and mental balance	Used in aromatherapy to uplift and harmonize
7. Respiratory System	Supports lung health and relieves congestion	Expectorant and antibacterial action

Precautions

- Generally non-toxic and non-irritant.
- Always dilute for topical application (1–2%).
- Avoid contact with eyes and sensitive areas.
- Store in dark, cool bottles away from sunlight.

7.27 Peppermint Essential Oil

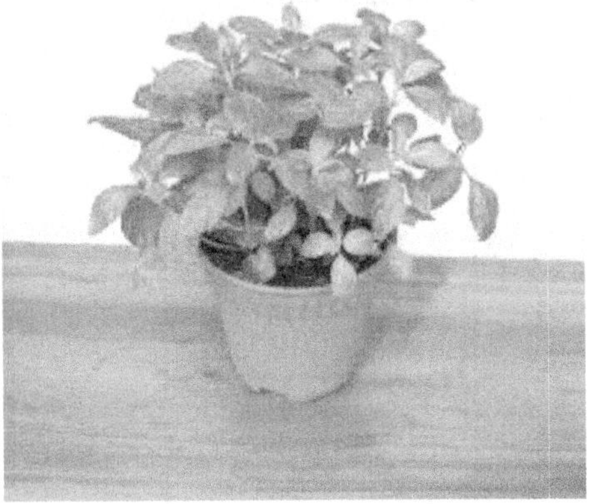

Introduction

Peppermint essential oil is a cooling, minty, and refreshing oil extracted from the leaves of *Mentha × piperita*. It is widely used in aromatherapy, digestive care, respiratory health, and pain relief due to its antispasmodic, analgesic, antimicrobial, and invigorating properties.

Botanical Source

- Botanical Name: *Mentha × piperita*
- Family: *Lamiaceae*
- Common Name: Peppermint
- Part Used: Leaves and flowering tops
- Origin: Hybrid of watermint and spearmint; native to Europe; cultivated worldwide

Physical & Chemical Properties

- Color: Clear to pale yellow
- Odor: Strong, fresh, minty, penetrating
- Consistency: Thin
- Perfumery note: Top note
- Main chemical constituents:
- Menthol (35–50%)
- Menthone
- 1,8-Cineole
- Limonene
- Menthyl acetate

Therapeutic Properties

- Carminative – Relieves gas and bloating
- Antispasmodic – Reduces cramps
- Analgesic – Pain relieving
- Antiemetic – Relieves nausea
- Expectorant – Clears respiratory tract
- Antimicrobial – Fights bacteria
- Cooling & refreshing – Stimulates mind

Therapeutic Uses

Digestive System

- Indigestion
- Flatulence
- Nausea & vomiting
- Irritable bowel

Respiratory System

- Cold
- Sinusitis
- Asthma
- Nasal congestion

Nervous System

- Mental fatigue
- Headache
- Migraine
- Lack of concentration

Musculoskeletal System

- Muscle pain
- Joint pain
- Sprains

Aromatherapy Applications

- Inhalation: For headache and sinus congestion
- Massage oil: 1–2% dilution for muscle pain
- Abdominal massage: For indigestion
- Foot bath: For tired feet
- Compress: For fever (cooling effect)

Safety & Precautions

- Avoid in children below 6 years
- Avoid during pregnancy (first trimester)
- Do not apply near eyes
- Can cause skin irritation – dilute properly (1–2%)
- Avoid in G6PD deficiency and in infants
- Excess use may cause skin sensitization

Blending with Other Oils

Peppermint blends well with:

- Lavender
- Eucalyptus
- Rosemary
- Lemon
- Tea Tree

7.28 Patchouli Essential Oil

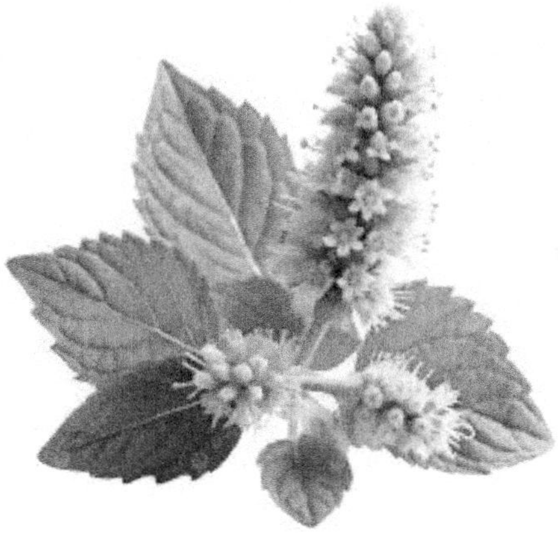

Introduction

Patchouli essential oil is a deep, earthy, musky oil extracted from the leaves of *Pogostemon cablin*. It is widely used in aromatherapy, perfumery, and skincare due to its grounding, calming, and skin-regenerative properties. Traditionally, it has been used for stress relief, emotional balance, and skin healing.

Botanical Source

- Botanical Name: *Pogostemon cablin*
- Family: *Lamiaceae*
- Common Name: Patchouli
- Part Used: Dried leaves
- Origin: Native to Southeast Asia; cultivated in Indonesia, Philippines, and India

Extraction Method

- Method: *Steam Distillation*
- Part Used: Dried leaves
- Yield: 1–3%
- Color: Dark amber to brown
- Aroma: Earthy, woody, musky, slightly sweet

Chemical Composition

Main constituents include:

- **Patchoulol (Patchouli alcohol)**
- **α-Bulnesene**
- **α-Guaiene**
- **α-Patchoulene**
- **Norpatchoulenol**

These compounds are responsible for its anti-inflammatory, antimicrobial, grounding, and regenerative effects.

Aromatic Profile

- Note: Base note
- Blends Well With: Bergamot, Lavender, Sandalwood, Rose, Orange, Vetiver

Therapeutic Benefits of Patchouli Essential Oil

System / Area	Therapeutic Benefits	Mechanism / Application
1. Nervous System	Reduces stress, anxiety, and depression	Grounding aroma stabilizes emotions and calms the mind
2. Skin Care	Heals scars, eczema, acne, and dry skin	Regenerative and antimicrobial properties
3. Immune System	Supports immunity and fights infections	Antimicrobial and antioxidant effects
4. Musculoskeletal System	Relieves muscle tension and joint pain	Anti-inflammatory and relaxing properties
5. Respiratory System	Eases colds and coughs	Mild expectorant and antimicrobial activity
6. Emotional & Spiritual Health	Promotes relaxation, meditation, and emotional balance	Used in aromatherapy for grounding and focus
7. Circulatory System	Improves blood flow	Stimulates circulation and lymphatic drainage

Precautions

- Generally safe when diluted (1–2%) for topical use.
- Avoid contact with eyes and sensitive areas.
- Use cautiously in pregnancy.
- Store in dark, cool bottles away from sunlight.

7.29 Pine Essential Oil

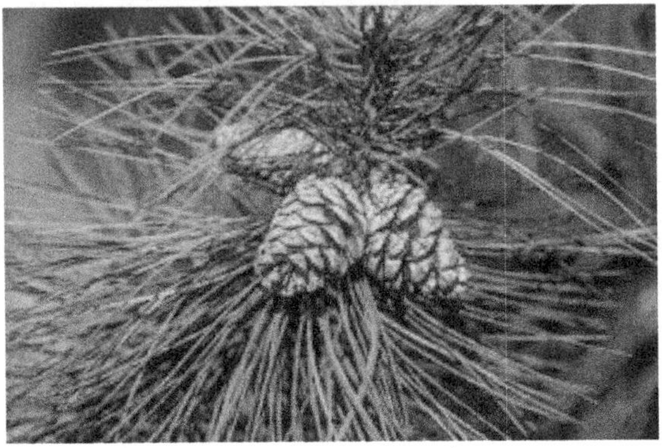

Introduction

Pine essential oil is a fresh, woody, and invigorating oil extracted from the needles and twigs of pine trees (*Pinus* species). It is widely used in aromatherapy, respiratory care, and household cleaning for its antimicrobial, anti-inflammatory, and decongestant properties. Pine oil helps refresh the mind, clear airways, and relieve muscle aches.

Botanical Source

- Botanical Name: *Pinus sylvestris* (Scotch Pine), *Pinus pinaster*, *Pinus ponderosa* (others)
- Family: *Pinaceae*
- Common Name: Pine
- Part Used: Needles, twigs, and sometimes resin
- Origin: Native to Europe, Asia, and North America; cultivated globally

Extraction Method

- Method: *Steam Distillation*
- Part Used: Fresh or partially dried needles and twigs
- Yield: 0.5–1%
- Color: Pale yellow to green
- Aroma: Fresh, woody, sharp, resinous

Chemical Composition

Main constituents include:

- α-Pinene (30–60%) – anti-inflammatory and bronchodilator
- β-Pinene
- Limonene
- Camphene
- Bornyl acetate

These compounds give pine oil its antimicrobial, anti-inflammatory, expectorant, and stimulating properties.

Aromatic Profile

- Note: Top note
- Blends Well With: Eucalyptus, Lavender, Rosemary, Lemon, Fir, Cedarwood

Therapeutic Benefits of Pine Essential Oil

System / Area	Therapeutic Benefits	Mechanism / Application
1. Respiratory System	Clears nasal congestion, relieves coughs, bronchitis	Expectorant and anti-inflammatory properties
2. Musculoskeletal System	Reduces muscle aches, joint pain, and stiffness	Anti-inflammatory and analgesic effects
3. Nervous System	Reduces mental fatigue and stress	Uplifting aroma stimulates CNS and enhances focus
4. Skin Care	Treats minor wounds, cuts, and oily skin	Antiseptic and astringent properties
5. Immune System	Supports immunity and fights infections	Antimicrobial and antioxidant effects
6. Circulatory System	Improves blood circulation and reduces fatigue	Stimulating and tonic effect
7. Household Uses	Natural disinfectant and deodorizer	Purifies air, repels insects, cleans surfaces

Precautions

- Avoid use in infants and sensitive skin.
- Should be diluted for topical application (1–2%).
- Avoid contact with eyes and mucous membranes.
- Use cautiously during pregnancy.

7.30 Rose Essential Oil

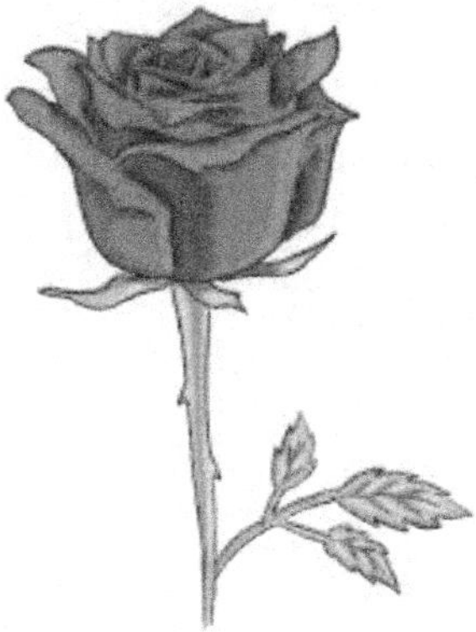

Introduction

Rose essential oil is a luxurious, sweet, and floral oil extracted from the petals of *Rosa* species. It is highly valued in aromatherapy, skincare, and perfumery for its emotional, anti-aging, and skin-regenerative properties. Traditionally, rose oil has been used to uplift mood, balance hormones, and rejuvenate skin.

Botanical Source

- Botanical Name: *Rosa damascena* (Damask rose), *Rosa centifolia* (Cabbage rose)
- Family: *Rosaceae*
- Common Name: Rose
- Part Used: Fresh petals
- Origin: Native to the Middle East; cultivated in Bulgaria, Turkey, India, and Iran

Extraction Method

- Method: *Steam Distillation* or *Solvent Extraction* (for absolute)
- Part Used: Fresh petals
- Yield: 0.02–0.05% (very low yield)
- Color: Pale yellow to deep amber (absolute)
- Aroma: Sweet, floral, rich, and uplifting

Chemical Composition

Main constituents include:

- Citronellol
- Geraniol
- Nerol
- Phenyl ethyl alcohol (PEA)
- Farnesol
- Eugenol (trace)

These compounds give rose oil its antidepressant, antimicrobial, anti-inflammatory, and skin-regenerative properties.

Aromatic Profile

- Note: Middle to top note
- Blends Well With: Lavender, Geranium, Sandalwood, Bergamot, Neroli, Patchouli

Therapeutic Benefits of Rose Essential Oil

System / Area	Therapeutic Benefits	Mechanism / Application
1. Nervous System	Reduces anxiety, depression, and emotional stress	Calming and uplifting aroma affects CNS
2. Skin Care	Heals scars, wrinkles, acne; hydrates and rejuvenates	Antioxidant, regenerative, anti-inflammatory
3. Hormonal & Reproductive Health	Balances hormones, relieves PMS and menstrual discomfort	Phytoestrogenic and relaxing properties
4. Immune System	Supports immunity and protects skin	Antimicrobial and antioxidant effects
5. Cardiovascular System	Lowers blood pressure and enhances circulation	Relaxing and tonic effect
6. Emotional & Spiritual Health	Enhances mood, meditation, and emotional clarity	Used in aromatherapy for stress relief
7. Respiratory System	Soothes respiratory irritation	Mild antimicrobial and anti-inflammatory properties

Precautions

- Generally safe when diluted (1–2%) for topical use.
- Avoid contact with **eyes and sensitive areas**.
- Store in **dark, cool bottles** away from sunlight.
- Pregnant women should use under medical supervision.

7.31 Rosemary Essential Oil

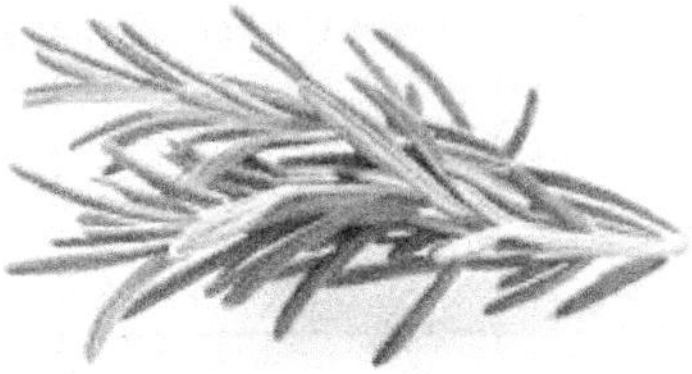

Introduction

Rosemary essential oil is a fresh, herbal, and woody oil extracted from the leaves and flowering tops of *Rosmarinus officinalis*. It is widely used in aromatherapy, hair care, cognitive support, and pain relief due to its stimulating, antioxidant, and antimicrobial properties. Rosemary oil is known to enhance memory, improve circulation, and relieve muscular pain.

Botanical Source

- Botanical Name: *Rosmarinus officinalis*
- Family: *Lamiaceae*
- Common Name: Rosemary
- Part Used: Leaves and flowering tops
- Origin: Native to the Mediterranean region; cultivated worldwide

Extraction Method

- Method: *Steam Distillation*
- Part Used: Fresh or dried leaves and flowering tops
- Yield: 1–2%
- Color: Pale yellow to green
- Aroma: Herbal, woody, fresh, slightly camphorous

Chemical Composition

Main constituents include:

- 1,8-Cineole (Eucalyptol)
- Camphor
- α-Pinene
- Borneol
- Verbenone

These compounds give rosemary oil its stimulating, antimicrobial, analgesic, and antioxidant properties.

Aromatic Profile

- Note: Middle to top note
- Blends Well With: Lavender, Peppermint, Lemon, Cedarwood, Thyme, Bergamot

Therapeutic Benefits of Rosemary Essential Oil

System / Area	Therapeutic Benefits	Mechanism / Application
1. Nervous System & Cognitive	Enhances memory, concentration, and mental clarity	Stimulates CNS and improves alertness
2. Hair & Scalp Care	Reduces dandruff, strengthens hair, promotes growth	Improves circulation, antimicrobial effect
3. Musculoskeletal System	Relieves muscle pain, arthritis, and stiffness	Analgesic and anti-inflammatory properties
4. Respiratory System	Clears congestion, relieves cough, asthma	Expectorant and decongestant activity
5. Digestive System	Improves digestion, reduces bloating	Stimulates digestive enzymes and smooth muscles
6. Skin Care	Reduces oily skin, acne, and minor wounds	Antimicrobial and astringent properties
7. Emotional & Mood	Reduces stress and mental fatigue	Uplifting and stimulating aroma

Precautions

- Avoid use in pregnancy, epilepsy, and sensitive skin.
- Dilute before topical use (1–2%).
- Avoid contact with eyes and mucous membranes.
- Store in dark glass bottles away.

7.32 Sandalwood Essential Oil

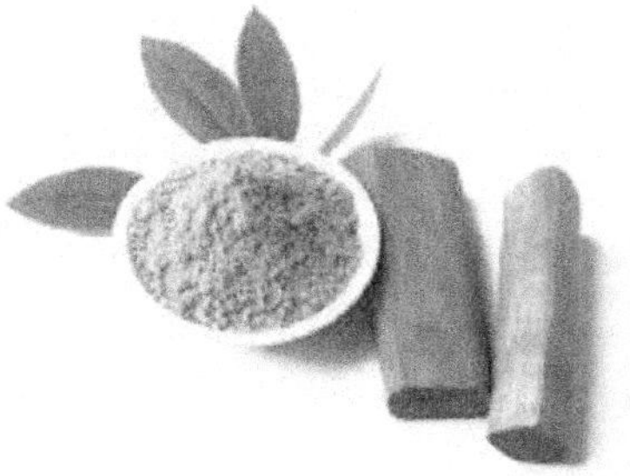

Introduction

Sandalwood essential oil is a rich, warm, woody oil extracted from the heartwood of *Santalum* species. Highly prized in aromatherapy, perfumery, and skincare, sandalwood oil is known for its calming, grounding, and regenerative properties. Traditionally, it has been used to relieve stress, improve mental clarity, and rejuvenate skin.

Botanical Source

- Botanical Name: *Santalum album* (Indian Sandalwood), *Santalum spicatum* (Australian Sandalwood)
- Family: *Santalaceae*
- Common Name: Sandalwood
- Part Used: Heartwood
- Origin: Native to India and Australia; cultivated in Indonesia and Hawaii

Extraction Method

- **Method:** *Steam Distillation*
- **Part Used:** Heartwood (dried)
- **Yield:** 3–8% (depending on quality)
- **Color:** Pale yellow to golden
- **Aroma:** Warm, woody, sweet, and long-lasting

Chemical Composition

Main constituents include:

- α-Santalol (40–55%)
- β-Santalol (15–20%)
- Santalenes
- α-Bisabolol
- Kaurene

These compounds are responsible for anti-inflammatory, antiseptic, sedative, and skin-regenerative properties.

Aromatic Profile

- Note: Base note
- Blends Well With: Rose, Lavender, Patchouli, Frankincense, Neroli, Bergamot

Therapeutic Benefits of Sandalwood Essential Oil

System / Area	Therapeutic Benefits	Mechanism / Application
1. Nervous System	Reduces anxiety, stress, and promotes mental clarity	Calming and grounding aroma affects CNS
2. Skin Care	Treats acne, scars, dry skin, and inflammation	Antiseptic, anti-inflammatory, and regenerative effects
3. Immune System	Supports immunity and protects against infections	Antimicrobial and antioxidant properties
4. Respiratory System	Relieves cough, cold, and congestion	Mild expectorant and soothing effect
5. Emotional & Spiritual Health	Enhances meditation, mental clarity, and emotional balance	Used in aromatherapy for grounding and focus
6. Anti-inflammatory & Pain Relief	Reduces muscle and joint pain	Anti-inflammatory and analgesic effects
7. Sleep & Relaxation	Improves sleep quality	Sedative and calming properties

Precautions

- Generally safe when diluted (1–2%) for topical use.
- Avoid contact with **eyes and sensitive areas**.
- Use high-quality, pure sandalwood oil for effectiveness.
- Store in **dark, cool bottles** away from sunlight.

7.33 Tarragon Essential Oil

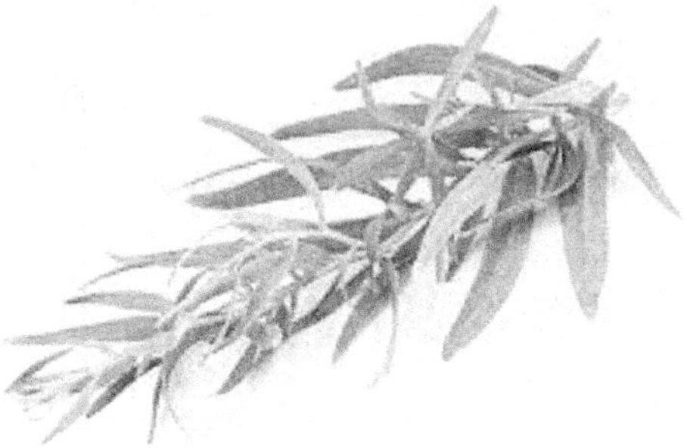

Introduction

Tarragon essential oil is a warm, sweet, and herbaceous oil extracted from the leaves and flowering tops of *Artemisia dracunculus*. Known for its digestive, anti-inflammatory, and calming properties, tarragon oil is widely used in aromatherapy, digestive support, and skincare. It has a slightly spicy and anise-like aroma, making it useful for both therapeutic and culinary applications.

Botanical Source

- Botanical Name: *Artemisia dracunculus*
- Family: *Asteraceae*
- Common Name: Tarragon
- Part Used: Leaves and flowering tops
- Origin: Native to Eurasia; cultivated in Europe, North America, and Asia

Extraction Method

- Method: *Steam Distillation*
- Part Used: Fresh or dried leaves and flowering tops
- Yield: 0.2–0.4%
- Color: Pale yellow
- Aroma: Sweet, herbaceous, slightly spicy, and anise-like

Chemical Composition

Main constituents include:

- Estragole (Methyl chavicol) – 60–75%
- Ocimene
- Methyl eugenol
- β-Phellandrene
- Caryophyllene

These compounds give tarragon oil its antimicrobial, anti-inflammatory, digestive, and calming properties.

Aromatic Profile

- Note: Middle note
- Blends Well With: Basil, Lavender, Lemon, Rosemary, Bergamot, Geranium

Therapeutic Benefits of Tarragon Essential Oil

System / Area	Therapeutic Benefits	Mechanism / Application
1. Digestive System	Relieves indigestion, bloating, gas, and poor appetite	Stimulates digestive enzymes and smooth muscles
2. Nervous System	Reduces anxiety, stress, and mental fatigue	Calming and balancing aroma promotes relaxation
3. Musculoskeletal System	Relieves muscle pain, cramps, and joint stiffness	Anti-inflammatory and antispasmodic properties
4. Circulatory System	Improves blood circulation	Vasodilatory and stimulating effect
5. Skin Care	Soothes minor skin irritation and inflammation	Anti-inflammatory and antimicrobial
6. Respiratory System	Supports respiratory health and eases congestion	Mild expectorant and anti-inflammatory action
7. Emotional & Mood	Enhances emotional balance and mental clarity	Used in aromatherapy to uplift and focus

Precautions

- Avoid during pregnancy and breastfeeding.
- Dilute before topical application (1–2%).
- Avoid use in individuals with sensitive skin or epilepsy.
- Store in dark, cool bottles away from sunlight

7.34 Tea Tree Essential Oil

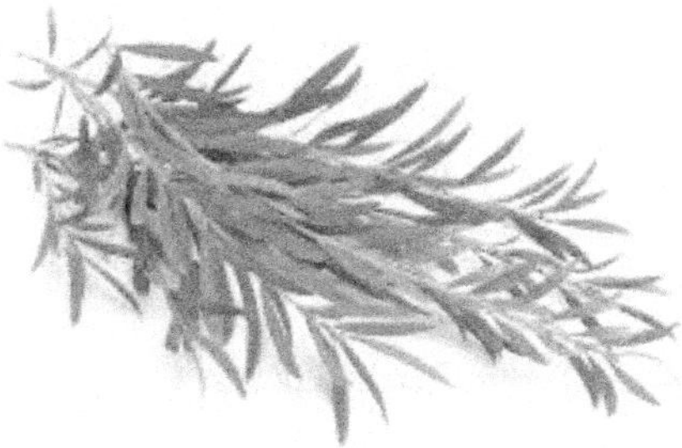

Introduction

Tea tree essential oil is a fresh, camphoraceous, medicinal oil extracted from the leaves of *Melaleuca alternifolia.* It is widely used in aromatherapy, skincare, and natural medicine for its antimicrobial, antifungal, antiviral, and anti-inflammatory properties. Tea tree oil is particularly effective for acne, wounds, infections, and respiratory support.

Botanical Source

- Botanical Name: *Melaleuca alternifolia*
- Family: *Myrtaceae*
- Common Name: Tea Tree
- Part Used: Leaves
- Origin: Native to Australia; cultivated in many parts of the world

Extraction Method

- Method: *Steam Distillation*
- Part Used: Fresh or partially dried leaves
- Yield: 1–3%
- Color: Pale yellow to light green
- Aroma: Fresh, medicinal, camphoraceous

Chemical Composition

Main constituents include:

- Terpinen-4-ol (30–40%) – antimicrobial & antifungal
- γ-Terpinene
- α-Terpinene
- 1,8-Cineole (Eucalyptol) – respiratory support
- α-Pinene

These compounds are responsible for **antimicrobial, anti-inflammatory, and antiseptic** properties.

Aromatic Profile

- Note: Top note
- Blends Well With: Lavender, Eucalyptus, Lemon, Rosemary, Peppermint, Tea Tree

Therapeutic Benefits of Tea Tree Essential Oil

System / Area	Therapeutic Benefits	Mechanism / Application
1. Skin Care	Treats acne, wounds, fungal infections, insect bites	Antimicrobial, antifungal, and anti-inflammatory properties
2. Immune System	Helps fight infections	Antibacterial, antiviral, antifungal effects
3. Respiratory System	Relieves congestion, coughs, and colds	Expectorant and antimicrobial action
4. Hair & Scalp	Reduces dandruff and lice	Antifungal and antibacterial
5. Musculoskeletal System	Relieves minor aches and inflammation	Anti-inflammatory and analgesic effects
6. Oral Health	Helps prevent gingivitis and bad breath	Antimicrobial and antiseptic
7. Emotional & Mood	Refreshing and uplifting	Stimulating aroma improves mental clarity

Precautions

- Generally safe when diluted (1–2%) for topical use.
- Avoid contact with eyes and mucous membranes.
- Avoid ingestion unless under professional supervision.
- Use with caution on sensitive skin and in children under 6 years.
- Store in dark, cool bottles away from sunlight.

7.35 Thyme Essential Oil

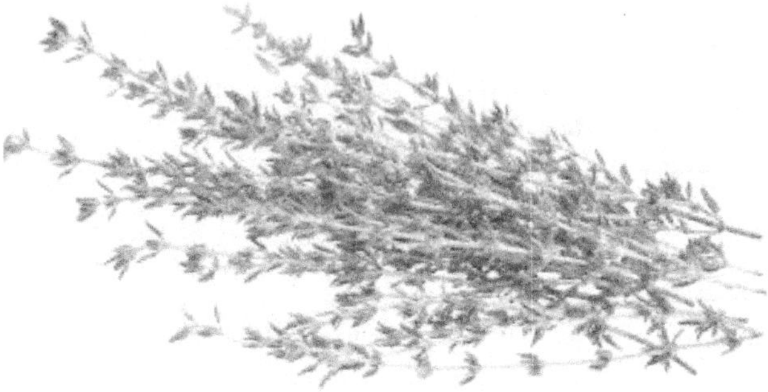

Introduction

Thyme essential oil is a herbal, warm, and slightly spicy oil extracted from the leaves and flowering tops of *Thymus vulgaris*. It is widely used in aromatherapy, respiratory care, and antimicrobial applications due to its antiseptic, antimicrobial, and anti-inflammatory properties. Thyme oil is effective in supporting immunity, respiratory health, and skin care.

Botanical Source

- Botanical Name: *Thymus vulgaris*
- Family: *Lamiaceae*
- Common Name: Thyme
- Part Used: Leaves and flowering tops
- Origin: Native to the Mediterranean region; cultivated worldwide

Extraction Method

- Method: *Steam Distillation*
- Part Used: Fresh or partially dried leaves and flowering tops
- Yield: 1–2%
- Color: Pale yellow to green
- Aroma: Warm, herbaceous, slightly spicy

Chemical Composition

Main constituents include:

- Thymol – 20–60% (antimicrobial, antioxidant)
- Carvacrol – 5–15% (antibacterial, antifungal)
- p-Cymene
- γ-Terpinene
- Linalool

These compounds give thyme oil its antimicrobial, antioxidant, and anti-inflammatory properties.

Aromatic Profile

- Note: Top to middle note
- Blends Well With: Rosemary, Lavender, Lemon, Eucalyptus, Peppermint, Bergamot

Therapeutic Benefits of Thyme Essential Oil

System / Area	Therapeutic Benefits	Mechanism / Application
1. Respiratory System	Relieves cough, cold, bronchitis, and congestion	Expectorant, antimicrobial, and anti-inflammatory
2. Immune System	Fights infections and boosts immunity	Antimicrobial and antiviral properties
3. Skin Care	Treats acne, wounds, and fungal infections	Antiseptic, anti-inflammatory, and antimicrobial
4. Musculoskeletal System	Relieves muscle aches and joint pain	Anti-inflammatory and analgesic effects
5. Digestive System	Improves digestion and relieves bloating	Stimulates digestive enzymes and smooth muscles
6. Emotional & Mood	Reduces fatigue and improves mental clarity	Stimulating and uplifting aroma
7. Circulatory System	Improves blood circulation	Vasodilatory and tonic effect

Precautions

- Avoid direct application without dilution (1– 2%).
- Can irritate sensitive skin; always perform a patch test.
- Avoid use in pregnancy or by individuals with epilepsy.
- Store in dark, cool bottles away from sunlight.

7.36 Vetiver Essential Oil

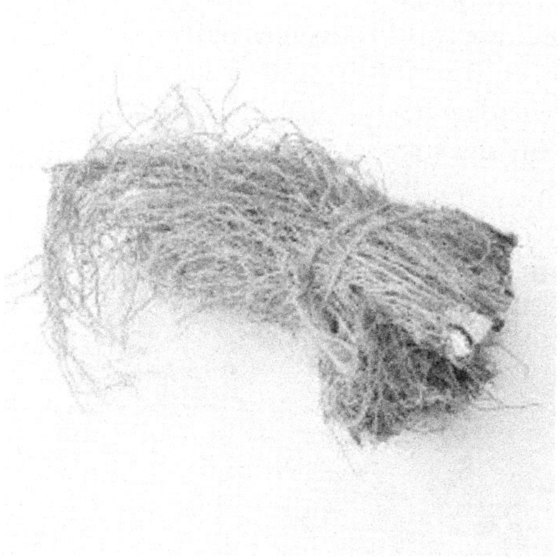

Introduction

Vetiver essential oil is a deep, earthy, woody oil extracted from the roots of *Vetiveria zizanioides*. It is renowned in aromatherapy, perfumery, and skincare for its calming, grounding, and rejuvenating properties. Traditionally, vetiver oil has been used to reduce stress, improve sleep, balance emotions, and promote healthy skin.

Botanical Source

- Botanical Name: *Vetiveria zizanioides*
- Family: *Poaceae*
- Common Name: Vetiver, Khus
- Part Used: Roots
- Origin: Native to India; also cultivated in Indonesia, Haiti, and Reunion Island

Extraction Method

- Method: *Steam Distillation*
- Part Used: Mature roots (10–18 months old)
- Yield: 0.5–1%
- Color: Dark brown to amber
- Aroma: Earthy, woody, smoky, deep, and grounding

Chemical Composition

Main constituents include:

- Vetiverol
- α-Vetivone
- β-Vetivone
- Khusimol
- Isovalencenol

These compounds give vetiver oil its sedative, anti-inflammatory, antioxidant, and regenerative properties.

Aromatic Profile

- Note: Base note
- Blends Well With: Lavender, Patchouli, Sandalwood, Bergamot, Rose, Frankincense

Therapeutic Benefits of Vetiver Essential Oil

System / Area	Therapeutic Benefits	Mechanism / Application
1. Nervous System & Emotional Health	Reduces stress, anxiety, depression; promotes emotional balance	Calming, grounding aroma affects CNS and stabilizes mood
2. Sleep & Relaxation	Improves sleep quality and reduces insomnia	Sedative and relaxing effect
3. Skin Care	Heals scars, burns, acne, and dry skin	Regenerative, anti-inflammatory, and antimicrobial properties
4. Musculoskeletal System	Relieves muscle tension, cramps, and joint pain	Anti-inflammatory and analgesic properties
5. Immune System	Supports immunity and prevents infections	Antimicrobial and antioxidant effect
6. Circulatory System	Enhances blood circulation and reduces fatigue	Stimulating and tonic effect
7. Meditation & Spiritual Health	Promotes grounding and mindfulness	Used in aromatherapy and meditation practices

Precautions

- Generally safe when diluted (1–2%) for topical use.
- Avoid contact with eyes and sensitive areas.
- Store in dark, cool bottles away from sunlight.
- Use high-quality, pure vetiver oil for best effects.

7.37 Ylang Ylang Essential Oil

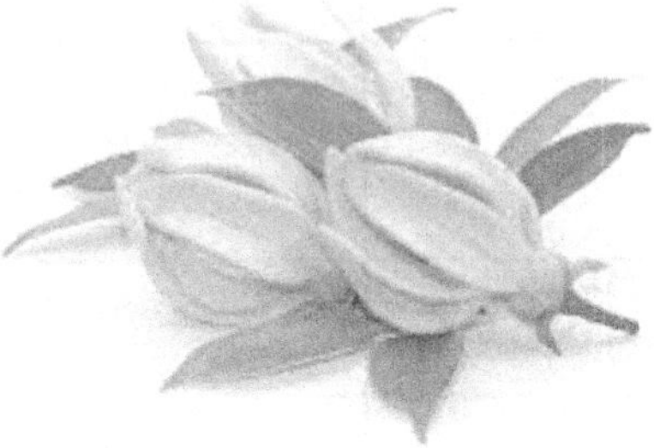

Introduction

Ylang Ylang essential oil is a sweet, floral, and exotic oil extracted from the flowers of *Cananga odorata*. It is widely used in aromatherapy, perfumery, and skincare for its calming, mood-enhancing, and aphrodisiac properties. Ylang Ylang oil is traditionally used to reduce stress, regulate heart rate, balance oil production in skin and hair, and enhance emotional well-being.

Botanical Source

- Botanical Name: *Cananga odorata*
- Family: *Annonaceae*
- Common Name: Ylang Ylang
- Part Used: Fresh flowers
- Origin: Native to tropical Asia, especially the Philippines, Indonesia, and Madagascar

Extraction Method

- Method: *Steam Distillation*
- Part Used: Fresh flowers
- Yield: 0.5–2%

- Color: Pale yellow to greenish
- Aroma: Sweet, floral, rich, and exotic

Chemical Composition

Main constituents include:

- Linalool – calming, sedative
- Geranyl acetate – relaxing, uplifting
- Caryophyllene – anti-inflammatory
- Benzyl acetate – sedative, calming
- Methyl benzoate

These compounds contribute to antidepressant, antiseptic, anti-inflammatory, and calming effects.

Aromatic Profile

- Note: Middle to base note
- Blends Well With: Bergamot, Lavender, Patchouli, Sandalwood, Rose, Geranium

Therapeutic Benefits of Ylang Ylang Essential Oil

System / Area	Therapeutic Benefits	Mechanism / Application
1. Nervous System & Emotional Health	Reduces stress, anxiety, depression; promotes relaxation	Sedative, calming, and mood-lifting aroma
2. Cardiovascular System	Regulates blood pressure and heart rate	Vasodilatory and calming effect
3. Skin & Hair Care	Balances sebum, treats acne, enhances hair growth	Antimicrobial, antiseptic, and sebum-regulating
4. Reproductive & Sexual Health	Acts as aphrodisiac, enhances libido	Aromatherapeutic and relaxing effects
5. Respiratory System	Eases breathing and reduces congestion	Mild antimicrobial and soothing action
6. Musculoskeletal System	Relieves tension and muscle cramps	Anti-inflammatory and relaxing effect
7. Spiritual & Meditative Use	Enhances meditation, mindfulness, and emotional balance	Calming and grounding effect in aromatherapy

Precautions

- Generally safe when diluted (1–2%) for topical use.
- Avoid contact with eyes and sensitive skin.
- High doses may cause headache or nausea in sensitive individuals.
- Store in dark, cool bottles away from sunlight

Chapter 8
Carrier oils

8.1 Almond oil

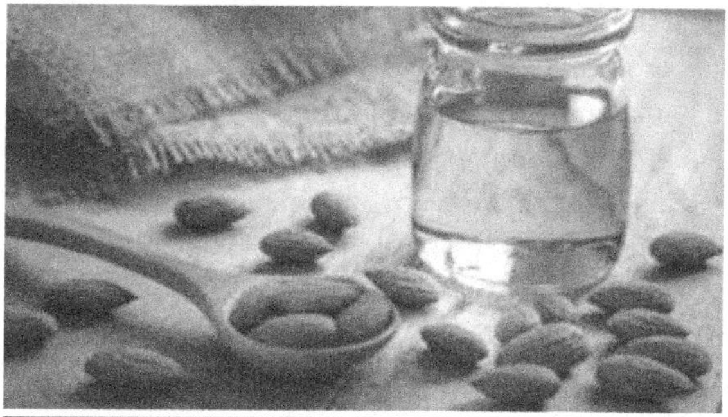

Introduction

Almond oil is a nutrient-rich plant oil extracted mainly from sweet almonds (*Prunus dulcis*) and is renowned for its wide range of health, cosmetic, and therapeutic uses. It is pale yellow in color, lightweight, and rapidly absorbed, making it an excellent moisturizer and massage oil for all skin types.

Origin and Extraction

Almond oil is derived from the kernels of almond trees, which originated in the Middle East and South Asia but are now grown worldwide, especially in the Mediterranean and California. Extraction methods like cold pressing help retain nutrients, while more modern processes (supercritical fluid and ultrasonic-assisted extraction) offer eco-friendly options and purity. Sweet almond oil is the most common for skin and cosmetic use, whereas bitter almond oil is only used for flavoring due to its natural toxins.

Composition and Nutritional Value

- Almond oil contains high levels of monounsaturated oleic acid (62–80%), linoleic acid (20–30%), and small amounts of saturated fats, mainly palmitic acid.
- It is rich in vitamin E (261% of daily value per 100ml), vitamin A, magnesium, phosphorus, and copper.
- Antioxidants like phytosterols and squalene contribute to its anti-inflammatory, skin-renewing, and cell-protective effects.

Health and Therapeutic Benefits

- Almond oil helps maintain healthy cholesterol and heart function by raising "good" HDL cholesterol and lowering "bad" LDL cholesterol and total cholesterol.
- It can boost immune function, aid in memory improvement, and potentially lower risks of cancer and heart disease.
- Used in traditional medicines (Ayurvedic, Chinese, and Greco-Persian), almond oil treats dry skin conditions, improves bowel transit, and supports overall skin health.

Cosmetic and Skin Applications

- Almond oil is highly emollient, which helps moisturize, balance water loss, and improve skin elasticity.
- It alleviates dryness, soothes skin irritations (eczema, psoriasis), lightens scars and stretch marks, and cleanses the skin as a gentle makeup remover.

- The oil's anti-inflammatory and antibacterial properties help prevent and treat acne and support skin barrier repair, making it suitable for sensitive skin and babies.
- It is also used as a massage oil, for aromatherapy, and for preventing fungal infections on the skin (e.g., athlete's foot).

Cooking Uses

- While sweet almond oil is sometimes used in cooking, its mild, nutty flavor makes it suitable for salad dressings and low-heat applications. Bitter almond oil, due to its toxicity, is only used for flavoring in minimal quantities.

Physical Properties

- Almond oil is pale yellow, non-volatile, and almost odorless, with a density of about 0.919g/ml.
- The oil is insoluble in water and highly soluble in organic solvents like chloroform or ether.

8.2. Apricot kernel oil

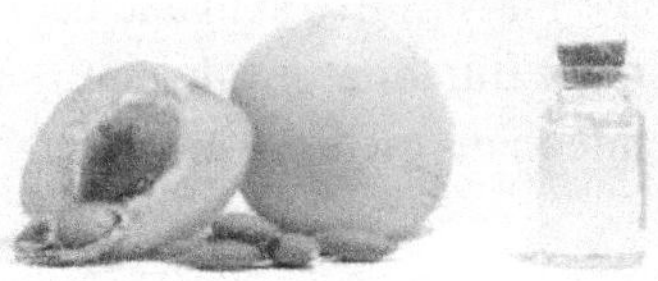

Apricot kernel oil is a light, quick-absorbing plant oil extracted from the seeds of apricots (*Prunus armeniaca*) and is especially valued in cosmetics and wellness routines for its gentle, nutrient-rich profile.

Chemical Composition and Nutrition

- Main constituents include oleic acid (57.9–68%), linoleic acid (22–30%), alpha-linolenic acid (omega-3, ~0.3%), palmitic acid (3–8%), stearic acid (1–2%), and palmitoleic acid (~1%).
- Rich in vitamin A, vitamin E (tocopherols ~50mg/100g), provitamin A (β-carotene ~61mg/g), and phytosterols (campesterol, stigmasterol, sitosterol).
- Contains polyphenols (caffeic acid, gallic acid, epicatechin, rutin, chlorogenic acid) and flavonoids (quercetin, catechins) which offer antioxidant, anti-inflammatory, and skin-protecting benefits.

Skin and Hair Benefits

- Intensely moisturizing: deeply softens and hydrates all skin types, especially mature, sensitive, or dry skin.

- Protects skin barrier, seals moisture, and smoothens texture for a glowing complexion—often found in face serums and creams.
- Reduces fine lines, wrinkles, and the appearance of dark circles due to its antioxidant content.
- Soothes acne, eczema, psoriasis, and other skin irritations by reducing inflammation and fighting bacteria.
- Boosts wound healing, collagen production, and skin regeneration.
- Used as a carrier oil for diluting essential oils, and in massage for easing joint and muscle pain.
- Promotes strong, healthy hair, moisturizes scalp, and reduces dandruff and hair loss.

Additional Benefits

- Antioxidant properties offer cell protection and combat environmental stress.
- Encourages blood circulation and may support heart health and immunity.
- Can be used for lip, nail, and cuticle care, and is sometimes added into food products for fortified nutrition.

Safety and Toxicity

- Sweet apricot kernel oil is safe for topical and dietary use; bitter varieties contain amygdalin, which can be toxic if consumed in large amounts, but sweet kernel oil is generally free of toxicity concerns.

Physical Properties

- Apricot kernel oil appears as a pale yellow liquid, is nearly odorless, and stands out for its light texture and rapid skin absorption.

8.3 Avacado Oil

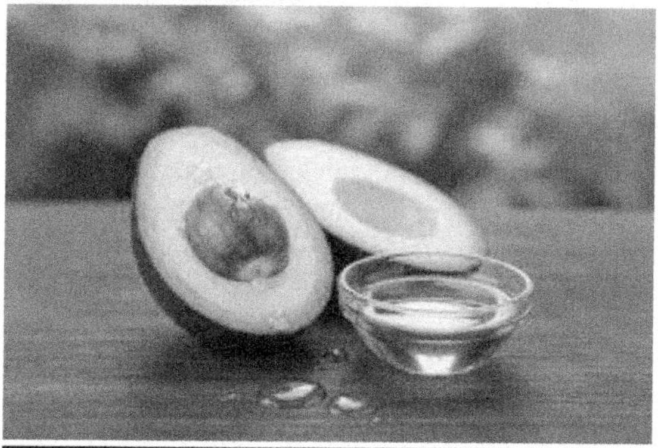

Introduction

Avocado oil is a highly nutritious, plant-based oil extracted from the pulp of the avocado fruit (*Persea americana*). Renowned for both culinary and cosmetic use, it is celebrated for its rich content of healthy fats, antioxidants, vitamins, and its beneficial effects on heart, skin, and overall wellness.

Composition and Nutritional Value

- Avocado oil is predominantly composed of monounsaturated fats, especially oleic acid (ranging from 50–70%), with smaller amounts of palmitic, palmitoleic, linoleic, and linolenic acids.
- One tablespoon contains:
- 124 calories
- 14 grams total fat (9.9g monounsaturated, 1.9g polyunsaturated, 1.6g saturated)
- No carbohydrates, fiber, or protein
- Contains vitamin E (tocopherol), lutein (a carotenoid important for eye health), beta-sitosterol, and phytosterols, which offer powerful antioxidant effects.

Health Benefits

- Supports heart health by lowering LDL ("bad") cholesterol and raising HDL ("good") cholesterol, much like olive oil.
- Rich in antioxidants (including vitamin E and lutein), which protect cells from oxidative stress and inflammation, and support skin and eye health.
- Aids absorption of fat-soluble vitamins A, D, E, and K when included in meals.
- May support healthy blood pressure and vascular function due to its beneficial fatty acid profile.
- High smoke point (~250°C/482°F) makes it suitable for frying, grilling, and various cooking methods without losing nutritional value.

Cosmetic and Skin Care Uses

- Used as a natural moisturizer and emollient for dry or sensitive skin, reducing inflammation and promoting smooth, hydrated skin.
- Common ingredient in creams, lotions, soaps, sunscreens, and hair care products for its ability to nourish, soothe, and protect skin and hair.
- Promotes wound healing, improves elasticity, and relieves skin conditions like eczema and psoriasis.

Physical and Organoleptic Properties

- Avocado oil is light yellow to yellowish-green (depending on refining), nearly odorless when refined but with a mild, buttery aroma and flavor in its unrefined, cold-pressed form.

- Liquid at room temperature and features a smooth, non-greasy texture.

Other Features

- Avocado oil is one of the few edible oils not derived from seeds but rather from the fruit's pulp.
- Its stable monounsaturated fats make it less likely to oxidize, offering better shelf life and usage for high-heat cooking.

8.4 Carrot Oil

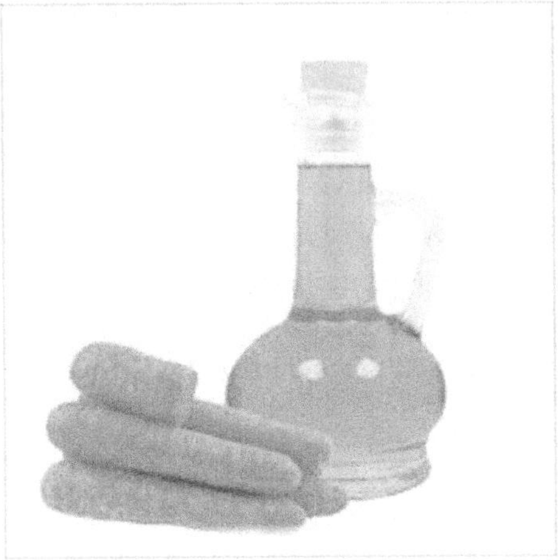

Carrot oil (commonly referring to carrot seed oil) is a nutrient-rich essential or carrier oil extracted from the seeds of the carrot plant (*Daucus carota*), prized for its potent antioxidant, anti-inflammatory, and skin-rejuvenating properties.

Composition and Nutritional Value

- Contains carotenoids (notably beta-carotene), vitamin A, vitamin E, potassium, and essential fatty acids like omega-6 linoleic acid and omega-9 oleic acid.
- Rich in flavones such as luteolin and its derivatives, and pharmacologically significant compounds like carotol and alpha-pinene, providing antioxidant, antibacterial, and anti-inflammatory effects.

Skin and Hair Benefits

- Potent antioxidant protects against free radical damage, slows aging, and helps maintain skin elasticity.
- Soothes, hydrates, and repairs dry, cracked, or irritated skin, improving skin tone and reducing fine lines and wrinkles.
- Alleviates skin disorders such as eczema, psoriasis, acne scars, and hyperpigmentation; also supports healing of minor sun damage due to compounds that absorb UVB light (not a sunscreen substitute).
- Promotes hair growth and health by strengthening the scalp, preventing hair loss, adding shine, and conditioning dry, frizzy hair.
- Used in creams, serums, soaps, and sun care products, and often added for extra nourishment in lip, beard, and nail care.

Additional Health and Therapeutic Benefits

- Antibacterial effects help in fighting *Staphylococcus aureus*, *Listeria monocytogenes*, and some fungal and yeast strains like *Candida*.
- Anti-inflammatory properties assist in soothing inflammation in skin and joints, and support general immune system health.
- Mild gastroprotective action and potential liver protection demonstrated in animal studies.

Physical Properties

- Carrot seed oil is typically light yellow to amber or pale orange-brown in color, with a woody, earthy, slightly sweet aroma.
- The carrier oil is non-greasy, absorbs well into the skin, and is intensely nourishing for mature, dry, and sun-damaged skin.

Safety and Usage

- Should be blended with a carrier oil (coconut, almond, grapeseed) before topical application due to possible skin sensitivity.
- Cold-pressed and steam distilled versions are available, each with slightly different profiles (essential oil for aromatherapy, carrier oil for skin/hair care).

8.5 Corn Oil

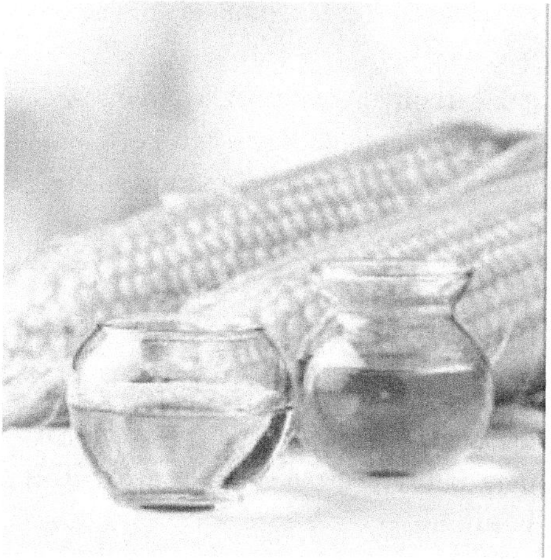

Introduction

Corn oil is a widely used edible vegetable oil extracted from the germ of corn (maize) kernels. It is known for its high polyunsaturated fat content, cholesterol-lowering potential, and various culinary and industrial uses.

Composition and Nutritional Value

- Corn oil is almost entirely composed of fat: about 99% triacylglycerols.
- In 100 grams, it provides:
    - 900 kcal
    - 100 g total fat (13 g saturated, 28 g monounsaturated, 55 g polyunsaturated)

    - 14 mg Vitamin E (nearly 95% of the daily value in a tablespoon)
- Rich in linoleic acid (omega-6, 53–59%), oleic acid (omega-9, 24–28%), and small amounts of alpha-linolenic acid (omega-3).
- Contains no protein, carbohydrates, fiber, vitamins A or C, or minerals, but it is high in phytosterols (8,300–25,500 ppm), especially beta-sitosterol, and tocopherols (1,130–1,830 ppm), both beneficial for health.

Health Benefits

- Corn oil's high polyunsaturated fat levels (especially omega-6 linoleic acid) help lower "bad" LDL cholesterol and may boost heart health when used in place of saturated or trans fats.
- The significant phytosterols and vitamin E content provide antioxidant and anti-inflammatory protection.
- It is easily digestible and provides energy and essential fatty acids that support skin health, cellular membranes, immune function, and production of important signaling molecules (icosanoids).

Culinary and Industrial Uses

- Corn oil's mild flavor and high smoke point make it ideal for deep frying, sautéing, baking, salad dressings, and margarine.
- Also found in processed foods, cosmetics, soaps, and as a carrier in some pharmaceuticals.
- Used in industrial applications for lubricants and plasticizers.

Considerations & Drawbacks

- Very high omega-6 content can imbalance the dietary ratio of omega-6 to omega-3 fatty acids if consumed excessively, which may promote inflammation.
- Nearly no micronutrients aside from vitamin E and phytosterols.
- Should be balanced with omega-3-rich foods in the diet.

Physical Properties

- Clear, pale yellow liquid with a neutral flavor and odor; stable for storage when refined.
- Commercially available in plastic jugs or bottles for home and industrial use

8.6 Primrose Oil

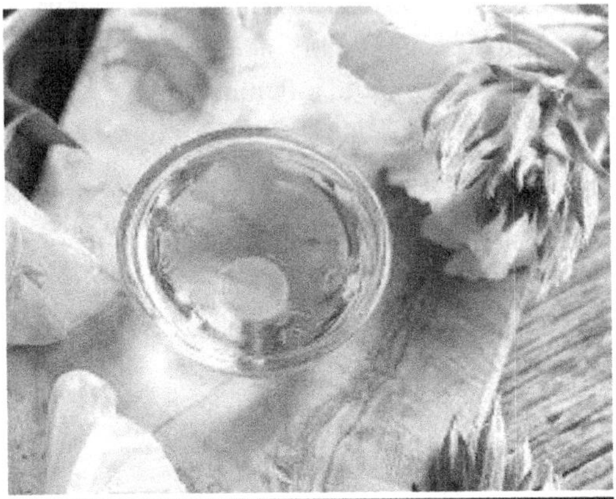

Introduction

Evening primrose oil (EPO) is a nutrient-rich oil extracted from the seeds of the evening primrose plant (*Oenothera biennis*), renowned for its high content of essential fatty acids, particularly linoleic acid and gamma-linolenic acid (GLA), which play key roles in anti-inflammatory and skin health benefits.

Composition and Nutritional Profile

- Contains approximately 74% linoleic acid (an omega-6 essential fatty acid), 9-10% gamma-linolenic acid (GLA), and smaller amounts of oleic acid (around 7%), palmitic acid, and stearic acid.
- Includes small quantities of tocopherols (vitamin E forms including alpha-, gamma-, and delta-tocopherols), triterpenes such as β-amyrin, squalene,

phenolic acids, phytosterols, and aliphatic alcohols, all contributing antioxidants and supportive compounds.

- Seeds also contain proteins, amino acids, minerals (calcium, potassium, magnesium), and vitamins A, B, C, and E.

Health Benefits and Therapeutic Uses

- The vital gamma-linolenic acid (GLA) in EPO is converted in the body to anti-inflammatory prostaglandins (such as prostaglandin E1), which support immune function, hormonal balance, and inflammation regulation.
- Commonly used as a dietary supplement to alleviate symptoms associated with premenstrual syndrome (PMS), menopausal discomfort, eczema, and other inflammatory skin conditions.
- Evidence suggests potential benefits for nerve damage in diabetes and osteoporosis when used alongside other nutrients, though more research is needed.
- Antioxidant properties help soothe dry, irritated skin and manage chronic skin inflammation such as eczema and psoriasis.

Usage and Safety

- EPO is consumed orally as softgels or capsules and applied topically for skin benefits.
- Generally regarded as safe at typical dosages but can cause mild side effects such as gastrointestinal upset or headaches in some individuals.
- Not a substitute for conventional treatments and scientific support is limited for many claimed uses.

Physical Characteristics

- Evening primrose oil is typically yellow to pale amber liquid with a light, nutty aroma.
- It has a light texture and is absorbable when used topically, often incorporated into skincare products for moisturizing and anti-inflammatory effects.

8.7 Grapeseed Oil

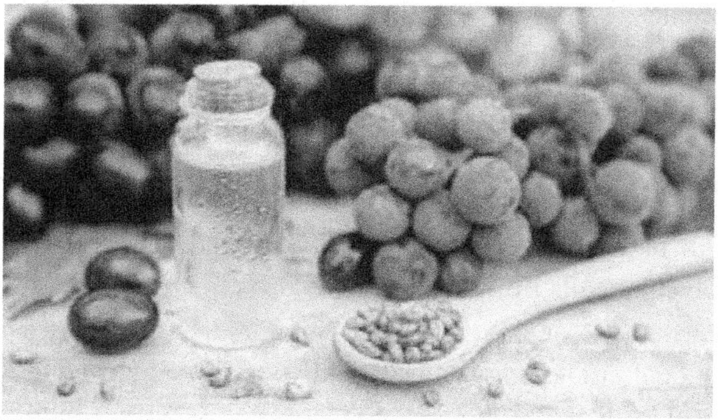

Introduction

Grapeseed oil is a light, versatile oil extracted from the seeds of grapes (*Vitis vinifera*), a byproduct of winemaking. It is valued for its high polyunsaturated fat content, vitamin E richness, and antioxidant properties, making it popular in culinary, cosmetic, and health applications.

Composition and Nutritional Profile

- Nutritional values per tablespoon:
    - Calories: 120
    - Total fat: 13.6 g (Saturated fat: 1.3 g, Monounsaturated fat: 2.2 g, Polyunsaturated fat: 9.5 g)
    - Vitamin E: 3.92 mg (19% of daily value)
    - Zero carbohydrates, sugars, protein, cholesterol, or sodium.
- Fatty acid composition is mainly polyunsaturated fats (~70%), predominantly linoleic acid (omega-6),

followed by monounsaturated fats (oleic acid) and some saturated fats.

- Contains plant phenolic antioxidants, including proanthocyanidins, which contribute to its anti-inflammatory and antioxidant potential.

Health Benefits

- High in vitamin E, which acts as a potent antioxidant protecting cells from damage.
- Rich linoleic acid content may support heart health by reducing LDL cholesterol and possibly improving vessel function, though concerns exist over high omega-6 intake relative to omega-3s.
- Anti-inflammatory and antioxidant properties have potential benefits for skin health, wound healing, and reducing oxidative stress.
- It is a common ingredient in skin and hair care products, where it moisturizes, protects, and promotes repair.

Culinary Uses

- Grapeseed oil has a mild, neutral flavor and a high smoke point (~216°C or 420°F), making it suitable for frying, sautéing, baking, and salad dressings.
- Often used as a substitute for other vegetable oils due to its light taste.

Physical Properties

- Clear, light yellow to greenish-yellow liquid with a subtle aroma.
- Derived as an extract from grape seeds left after wine production, making it a sustainable byproduct.

8.8 Hazelnut Oil

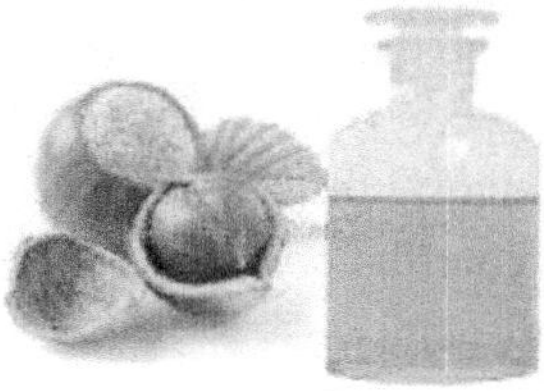

Introduction

Hazelnut oil is an edible oil extracted from the kernels of hazelnuts (*Corylus avellana*), highly prized for its rich nutritional profile dominated by healthy fats, vitamin E, and antioxidant compounds. It is widely used in culinary applications and skin care for its moisturizing and protective properties.

Composition and Nutritional Value

- Hazelnut oil contains approximately 50-73% oil by weight in the nut kernels, with the oil itself rich in monounsaturated fats (70-85% oleic acid), followed by polyunsaturated fats (10-20% linoleic acid) and a small amount of saturated fats (around 7-10% palmitic and stearic acids).

- One tablespoon (13.6 g) of hazelnut oil provides about 120 calories, mostly from fats, with negligible protein or carbohydrates.
- It is a rich source of vitamin E (α-tocopherol), providing around 6.4 mg per tablespoon, which covers approximately 42% of the recommended daily allowance (RDA).
- Contains phytosterols like sitosterol, campesterol, and delta-5-avenasterol, which contribute to cardiovascular benefits and cholesterol management.
- Rich in phenolic compounds such as flavonoids (catechin, epicatechin), phenolic acids (caffeic, ferulic, gallic acids), and stilbenes like resveratrol that add antioxidant and anti-inflammatory effects.

Health Benefits

- High oleic acid content supports cardiovascular health by reducing LDL cholesterol, improving lipid profiles, and offering anti-inflammatory effects.
- Vitamin E and phenolic antioxidants confer skin protective benefits, helping with anti-aging, skin repair, and UV protection, making it a popular ingredient in cosmetics.
- Phytosterols in the oil contribute to lowering cholesterol and supporting heart health.
- Hazelnut oil is suitable for people managing diabetes, as studies suggest benefits for blood sugar regulation and risk reduction for heart disease.

Culinary and Cosmetic Uses

- The oil has a mild, nutty flavor and aroma, making it ideal for salad dressings, sauces, drizzling, and light cooking.

- High smoke point (~430°F or 221°C) allows for versatile cooking applications.
- Frequently used topically for skin and hair care, providing deep moisturization and helping with dry or damaged skin and hair.

Physical Appearance

- Hazelnut oil is typically clear and golden yellow in color, with a smooth texture and pleasant nutty aroma.

8.9 Jojoba Oil

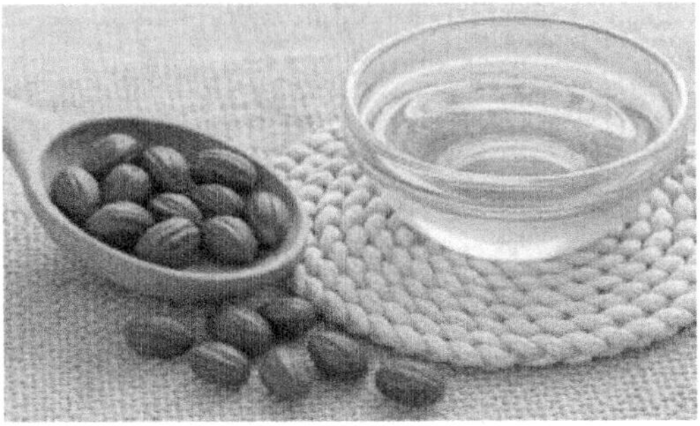

Jojoba oil is a unique plant-based liquid wax extracted from the seeds of the jojoba shrub (*Simmondsia chinensis*), native to arid regions. Its chemical composition closely resembles human skin sebum, making it highly compatible for skin and hair care.

Chemical Composition and Nutritional Profile

- Unlike typical oils composed mainly of triglycerides, jojoba oil consists of over 98% wax esters, made up of long-chain monohydric alcohols and fatty acids.
- Major fatty acids and alcohols include eicosenyl eicosenoate, docosenyl eicosenoate, erucic acid (C22:1), 11-eicosenoic acid, and nervonic acid, contributing to its stability and skin benefits.
- Contains small amounts of free fatty acids (less than 1%), free alcohols, sterols (such as cholesterol), and antioxidant fat-soluble vitamins, predominantly vitamin E (around 50 mg/100 g).
- Jojoba oil has a high proportion of monounsaturated fats (~97.6%) with negligible saturated (1.0%) and polyunsaturated fats (0.3%).

Physical Properties

- Jojoba oil is typically clear or pale yellow with a faint characteristic odor.
- It has a freezing point between 7-10.6°C, a smoke point around 195°C, a refractive index of 1.465, and a specific gravity of 0.863 at 25°C.
- Known for being chemically stable and resistant to oxidation due to its wax ester composition and antioxidant content.

Health and Cosmetic Benefits

- Due to its similarity to human sebum, jojoba oil is an excellent natural moisturizer; it absorbs easily, balances skin oil production, and helps prevent dryness and irritation.
- It supports skin barrier function, retains water, and provides anti-inflammatory effects beneficial for sensitive or acne-prone skin.
- Rich in vitamin E, B vitamins, copper, and zinc, jojoba oil delivers antioxidant protection, promotes skin repair, and may reduce skin inflammation.
- Used extensively in skin, hair, and body care products for moisturizing, soothing, softening hair, and protecting against damage.
- Jojoba oil is non-comedogenic and suitable for all skin types, including sensitive and oily skin.
- Due to its chemical stability, it is an ideal carrier oil for essential oils in aromatherapy and massage.

Usage and Precautions

- Extracted primarily by cold pressing jojoba seeds.
- Stable on storage and gentle, with no serious side effects reported when used topically.
- Should be stored in cool, dark conditions to maximize shelf life.

8.10 Olive Oil

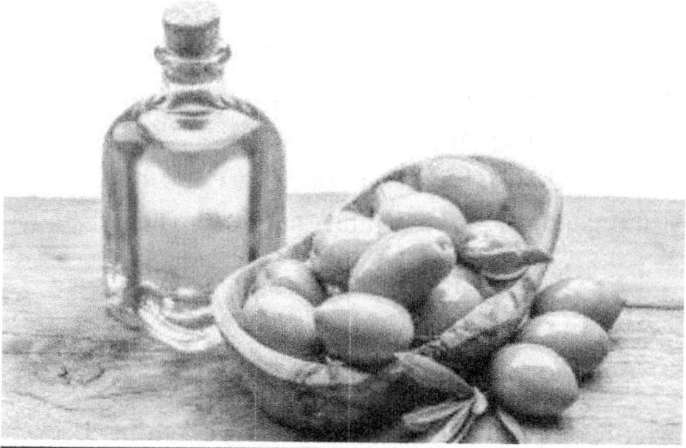

Introduction

Olive oil is a natural oil derived from the fruit of the olive tree (*Olea europaea*), widely esteemed for its rich composition of healthy fats, antioxidants, and bioactive compounds. It is a cornerstone of Mediterranean cuisine and a staple in health and beauty practices across the world.

Composition and Nutritional Value

- A tablespoon (about 14 grams) of extra virgin olive oil contains approximately 119 calories, predominantly from fats.
- Fat composition:
    - Monounsaturated fats (mostly oleic acid): about 73% of total calories
    - Saturated fat: about 14%
    - Polyunsaturated fat: about 11%

- Olive oil is a good source of vitamin E (about 13% of daily value per tablespoon) and vitamin K (about 7% of daily value).
- Contains powerful antioxidants such as oleocanthal and oleuropein, which exhibit anti-inflammatory and cardioprotective properties.
- The oleic acid predominant profile contributes to healthy cholesterol levels and supports heart and vascular health.

Health Benefits

- Regular consumption of extra virgin olive oil has been linked to reduced risks of cardiovascular disease through lowering LDL cholesterol and oxidative stress.
- The antioxidants in olive oil can help protect LDL cholesterol from oxidation, a risk factor for atherosclerosis.
- Olive oil has anti-inflammatory attributes that may contribute to protection against chronic diseases such as cancer, hypertension, and neurodegenerative disorders.
- It supports bone health, blood clotting, and overall metabolic health due to its vitamin K content.

Culinary Uses and Properties

- Olive oil is used for dressing salads, sautéing, frying, and as a finishing oil to lend flavor and health benefits to dishes.
- Extra virgin olive oil, known for minimal processing and high polyphenol content, is prized for its flavor and health qualities.
- It has a moderate smoke point (~190–220°C) suitable for most cooking methods, though delicate unrefined types are best for low-heat applications.

Physical Appearance and Historical Context

- Olive oil typically has a golden-yellow to greenish color, depending on the olive variety and processing.
- It has a rich, fruity aroma with slight bitterness and pepperiness in high-quality varieties.
- Olive oil production has ancient origins, with archaeological evidence of presses and oil extraction techniques dating back thousands of years.

8.11 Peanut Oil

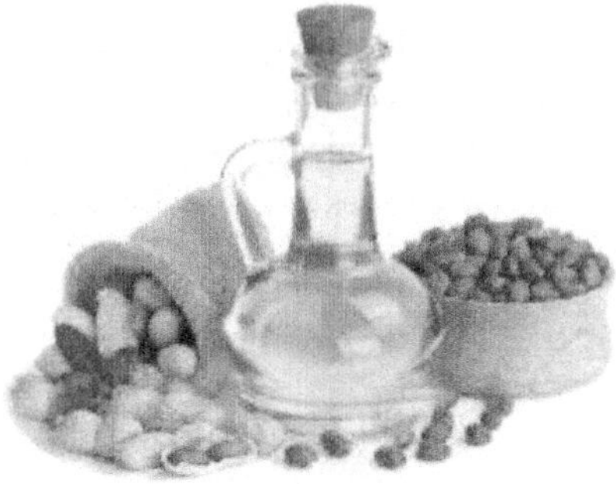

Introduction

Peanut oil, also known as groundnut oil, is an edible oil extracted from peanuts (*Arachis hypogaea*). It is widely used for cooking, frying, and in salad dressings due to its high smoke point and mild flavor. It is rich in healthy fats and antioxidants, making it beneficial for heart health and overall wellness.

Composition and Nutritional Profile

- Calories: Approximately 119-120 kcal per tablespoon (13.5g).
- Fat content: About 13.5 grams per tablespoon, consisting of:
    - Saturated fats: 2.3 grams
    - Monounsaturated fats: 6.2 grams

  - Polyunsaturated fats: 4.3 grams
  - Main fatty acids: oleic acid (omega-9), linoleic acid (omega-6).
- Vitamin E: Rich source, with about 14-16 mg per serving, acting as an antioxidant.
- Contains phytosterols, which support cholesterol reduction and cardiovascular health.

Health Benefits

- Heart health: The presence of monounsaturated and polyunsaturated fats along with vitamin E helps lower LDL cholesterol and protect against cardiovascular disease.
- Blood sugar regulation: Some studies suggest that replacing saturated fats with unsaturated fats from peanut oil can improve blood glucose levels, especially in people with diabetes.
- Antioxidant properties: Vitamin E contributes to reducing oxidative stress and inflammation, supporting overall cellular health.
- Skin and hair: Used topically, it nourishes skin, improves elasticity, and conditions hair.

Culinary Uses

- Suitable for deep frying, sautéing, roasting, and baking due to its high smoke point (~450°F or 232°C).
- Has a mild, nutty flavor that enhances a variety of recipes while retaining nutritional benefits.

Physical Characteristics

- Bright yellow color, with a smooth, light texture.
- Usually refined to remove impurities, but cold-pressed varieties retain more of the natural flavor and nutrients.

8.12 Safflower Oil

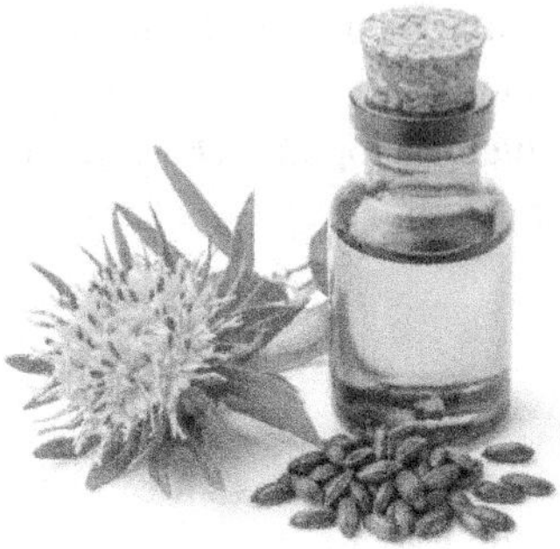

Introduction

Safflower oil is a vegetable oil extracted from the seeds of the safflower plant (*Carthamus tinctorius*). It is rich in unsaturated fatty acids, especially monounsaturated oleic acid and polyunsaturated linoleic acid, and is valued for its health benefits and culinary versatility.

Composition and Nutritional Profile

- Safflower oil contains approximately 884 kcal per 100 grams, with virtually no carbohydrates or protein.
- Fat content per 100 grams:
    - Total fats: 100 g
    - Saturated fat: 7.5 g
    - Monounsaturated fat: 75 g (primarily oleic acid)
    - Polyunsaturated fat: 13 g (primarily linoleic acid).

- Rich in vitamin E, providing about 102 mg per 100 grams (682% of the daily value).
- Contains vitamin K in smaller amounts (18% DV) and negligible quantities of other vitamins.

Health Benefits

- High in unsaturated fats, especially monounsaturated fats, which may help lower LDL cholesterol and promote cardiovascular health.
- The oil's vitamin E acts as a powerful antioxidant, reducing oxidative stress and inflammation.
- Its polyunsaturated fats support skin health, improve hydration, and may aid in managing conditions like eczema when used topically or consumed.
- Studies also investigate safflower oil's role in weight control and inflammation regulation, though conclusive evidence is limited.

Culinary Uses and Physical Characteristics

- Safflower oil has a mild flavor and high smoke point (~232°C or 450°F), making it suitable for frying, sautéing, baking, and salad dressings.
- It is clear to light yellow in appearance, commonly refined to improve stability and shelf life.

Botany and Oil Source

- Safflower oil is derived from the seeds of the safflower plant, which has bright orange to yellow spiny flower heads and green, bristly leaves.
- The seeds are rich in oil, which constitutes the primary commercial product harvested from safflower cultivation.

8.13 Sesame Oil

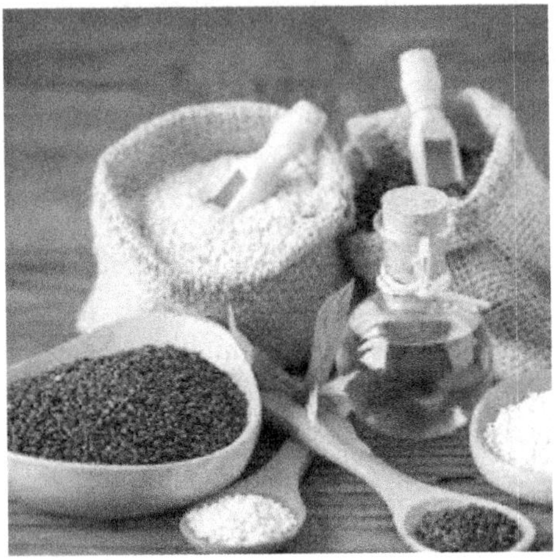

Introduction

Sesame oil is a highly valued edible and therapeutic oil extracted from the seeds of the sesame plant (*Sesamum indicum*). It has been used for thousands of years due to its rich nutritional profile, balanced fatty acid content, and potent antioxidant compounds.

Composition and Nutritional Profile

- Sesame oil provides about 120 calories per tablespoon (14g), composed entirely of fats with no protein or carbohydrates.
- Its fatty acid profile includes:
    - Monounsaturated fats (oleic acid): approximately 37-40%
    - Polyunsaturated fats (linoleic acid): approximately 42-45%

  - Saturated fats (mainly palmitic and stearic acid): around 5-7%.
- Rich in essential micronutrients such as vitamin E (tocopherols), providing about 25 mg/100 g, and vitamin K.
- Contains bioactive phytochemicals including lignans (sesamin, sesamolin), phytosterols, and antioxidants such as sesamol and sesamolinol, which contribute to its health-promoting properties.

Health Benefits

- Antioxidant compounds and vitamin E help reduce oxidative stress and inflammation.
- The balanced ratio of omega-6 to omega-9 fatty acids supports cardiovascular health by improving cholesterol levels and protecting blood vessels.
- Sesame oil demonstrates anti-inflammatory, antimicrobial, and possible anti-cancer effects, backed by preliminary research.
- Topical application aids in skin hydration, elasticity, and healing wounds; it is prized in traditional medicine for massage and dermatological uses.

Culinary Uses and Characteristics

- Sesame oil has a distinctive nutty aroma and light golden-yellow color, widely used in various cuisines, especially Asian dishes.
- It has a moderate smoke point (~210°C or 410°F), making it suitable for sautéing, stir-frying, and dressings.
- Unrefined sesame oil retains most phytochemicals and flavor, whereas refined oil has a neutral taste and lighter color

8.14 Soyabean Oil

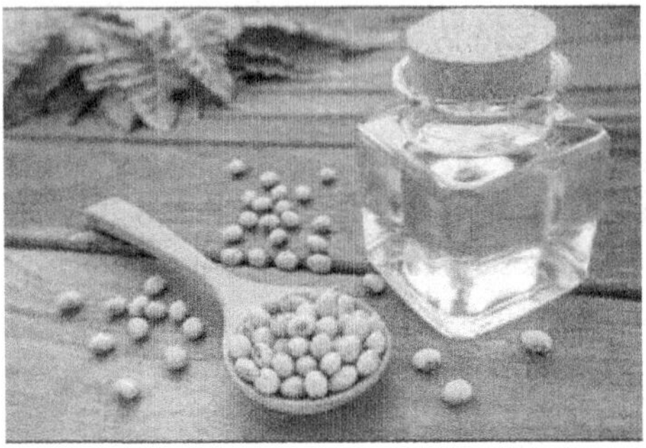

Introduction

Soybean oil is a widely consumed edible oil extracted from the seeds of the soybean plant (*Glycine max*), known for its high polyunsaturated fat content and nutritional value. It is commonly used in cooking, food manufacturing, and as a base for many processed foods.

Composition and Nutritional Profile

Soybean oil contains approximately:

- 12-15% saturated fat
- 22-30% monounsaturated fat (mainly oleic acid)
- 55-58% polyunsaturated fat (primarily linoleic acid and alpha-linolenic acid).

Key fatty acids:

- Linoleic acid (omega-6): ~50-55%
- Alpha-linolenic acid (omega-3): ~6-7%
- Oleic acid (omega-9): ~22-24%
- Palmitic acid (saturated): ~10-11%

- Stearic acid (saturated): ~4%

Contains important micronutrients such as vitamin E (tocopherols), predominantly γ- and δ-tocopherols, which contribute to antioxidant protection and oil stability.
Approximately 120 kcal per tablespoon, mainly from fats, with no carbohydrates or protein.

Health Benefits and Considerations

- Good source of essential fatty acids, including both omega-6 and omega-3, which support cardiovascular and overall health when balanced properly.
- Contains antioxidants which may reduce oxidative damage and inflammation.
- The omega-3 content (ALA) has benefits for heart and brain health; however, conversion to EPA and DHA in the body is limited.
- Excessive omega-6 intake in relation to omega-3 can promote inflammation, so a balanced diet is important.
- Used in many processed foods, salad dressings, mayonnaise, margarine, and cooking oils due to its neutral flavor and versatile use.

Physical Characteristics

- Soybean oil is a light yellow to golden liquid with a neutral taste and aroma, typically refined for cooking and food use.
- Cultivation of soybeans and processing of oil is widespread, especially in the US and South America, supporting large-scale production and use.

8.15 Sunflower Oil

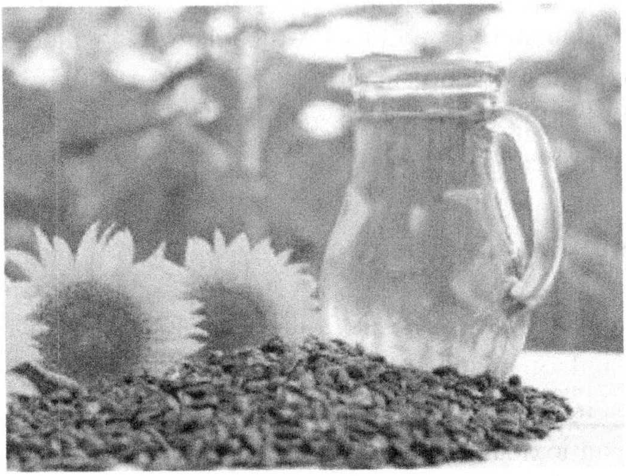

Introduction

Sunflower oil is a popular vegetable oil extracted from the seeds of the sunflower plant (*Helianthus annuus*). It is widely used worldwide in cooking, food production, and cosmetics because of its mild flavor, nutritional benefits, and versatile applications.

Composition and Nutritional Profile

- In 100 grams, sunflower oil provides approximately 900 kcal (3700 kJ), all from fats.
- Typical fatty acid profile:
  - Saturated fatty acids: 11-12 g
  - Monounsaturated fatty acids (mainly oleic acid): 24-27 g
  - Polyunsaturated fatty acids (mostly linoleic acid, omega-6): 62-64 g.

- Rich source of vitamin E, providing between 45 to 90 mg per 100 grams, which amounts to 375-750% of the recommended daily allowance.
- Variations in sunflower oil available commercially include:
    - High-linoleic (conventional): ~69% linoleic acid
    - High-oleic: up to 82% oleic acid
    - Mid-oleic and high-stearic variants, each with specific fatty acid balances.
- No cholesterol or carbohydrates are present.

Health Benefits

- Sunflower oil's high content of unsaturated fats, particularly polyunsaturated and monounsaturated fats, helps improve cholesterol levels and supports heart health.
- The oil's abundant vitamin E protects cells from oxidative damage and acts as a potent natural antioxidant.
- Studies show benefits in reducing inflammatory markers and potentially supporting skin health, due to its fatty acids and antioxidant content.

Culinary and Other Uses

- Suitable for frying, sautéing, baking, and salad dressings due to its mild flavor and high smoke point (~232°C or 450°F).
- Also used in cosmetics and skincare as an emollient and moisturizer.

Physical Characteristics

- Sunflower oil is light yellow to pale golden in color and clear in appearance.
- Variants exist based on fatty acid profiles due to plant breeding and processing methods.

Chapter-9
Contraindications of Aroma Oils

CONDITION	OILS TO BE AVOIDED
Pregnancy	Avoid *Clary Sage, Rosemary, Cinnamon, Basil, Juniper*—may stimulate uterine contractions
Infants & Children	Avoid *Peppermint, Eucalyptus, Wintergreen*—can cause respiratory distress or skin irritation
Epilepsy	Avoid *Fennel, Rosemary, Sage, Hyssop*—may trigger seizures due to neurotoxic compounds
High Blood Pressure	Avoid *Thyme, Rosemary, Hyssop*—can elevate blood pressure
Sensitive Skin / Allergies	Avoid *Cinnamon, Oregano, Lemongrass* undiluted—may cause burns, rashes, or allergic reactions
Asthma / Respiratory Issues	Avoid *strong camphoraceous oils* like Eucalyptus or Camphor—may worsen symptoms
Photosensitivity	Avoid *Citrus oils* (e.g., Bergamot, Lemon) before sun exposure—can cause skin burns
Pets (especially cats)	Avoid *Tea Tree, Citrus, Pine, Peppermint*—toxic to animals when inhaled or ingested

References

- Tisserand, R. & Young, R. (2014) – *Essential Oil Safety: A Guide for Health Care Professionals*
- Battaglia, S. (2003) – *The Complete Guide to Aromatherapy*
- National Center for Biotechnology Information (NCBI)
- Aromatherapy Science: A Guide for Healthcare Professionals – Maria Lis-Balchin
- Lawless, J. (2014). *The Encyclopedia of Essential Oils*. HarperCollins.
- Tisserand, R., & Young, R. (2014). *Essential Oil Safety: A Guide for Health Care Professionals*, 2nd Ed. Churchill Livingstone.
- Ali, B. et al. (2015). "Essential oils used in aromatherapy: A systematic review." *Asian Pacific Journal of Tropical Biomedicine*, 5(8): 601–611.
- Lis-Balchin, M. (2006). *Aromatherapy Science: A Guide for Healthcare Professionals*. Pharmaceutical Press.
- Koulivand, P.H. et al. (2013). "Lavender and Ylang-Ylang essential oils: A review on pharmacological effects and mechanisms." *Iranian Journal of Basic Medical Sciences*, 16(6): 752–759.
- Tisserand & Young (2014) – *Essential Oil Safety: A Guide for Health Care Professionals*
- The Complete Guide to Aromatherapy – Salvatore Battaglia
- National Association for Holistic Aromatherapy (NAHA)
- PubMed / NCBI studies on *Ocimum basilicum* pharmacological properties
- Chowdhury, A.R. et al. (2017). "Chemical composition and pharmacological activities of Vetiver (*Vetiveria zizanioides*) essential oil." *Journal of Essential Oil Research*, 29(5): 421–432.
- Battaglia, S. (2003) – *The Complete Guide to Aromatherapy*

- PubMed and NCBI for phytochemical studies on *Citrus bergamia*
- International Federation of Aromatherapists (IFA) guidelines
- Burt, S. (2004). "Essential oils: their antibacterial properties and potential applications in foods—a review." *International Journal of Food Microbiology*, 94(3): 223–253.
- Hammer, K.A., Carson, C.F., & Riley, T.V. (2002). "Antimicrobial activity of essential oils and other plant extracts." *Journal of Applied Microbiology*, 86(6): 985–990.
- Carson, C.F., Hammer, K.A., & Riley, T.V. (2006). "Melaleuca alternifolia (Tea Tree) oil: a review of antimicrobial and other medicinal properties." *Clinical Microbiology Reviews*, 19(1): 50–62.
- Dhiman, A. et al. (2018). "Chemical composition and biological activities of Tarragon (*Artemisia dracunculus*) essential oil." *Journal of Essential Oil Research*, 30(5): 333–340.
- Lawless, J. (2014). *The Encyclopedia of Essential Oils*. HarperCollins.
- Edris, A.E. (2007). "Pharmaceutical and therapeutic potentials of essential oils and their individual volatile constituents: a review." *Phytotherapy Research*, 21(4): 308–323.
- Carson, C.F., & Riley, T.V. (2003). "Antimicrobial activity of essential oils." *Clinical Microbiology Reviews*, 12(4): 564–582.
- Chidambara Murthy, K.N. et al. (2012). "Chemical composition and therapeutic properties of Indian Sandalwood (*Santalum album* L.) oil." *Journal of Essential Oil Research*, 24(6): 520–529.
- Perry, N. & Perry, E. (2006). "Aromatherapy in the management of psychiatric disorders." *CNS Drugs*, 20(4): 257–280.

- Cavanagh, H.M.A., & Wilkinson, J.M. (2002). "Biological activities of Rosemary essential oil." *Phytotherapy Research*, 16(4): 301–308.
- Perry, N.B., et al. (1999). "Essential oil composition of Rosemary (*Rosmarinus officinalis*) and its biological activity." *Journal of Agricultural and Food Chemistry*, 47(7): 2655–2660.
- Edris, A.E. (2007). "Pharmaceutical and therapeutic potentials of essential oils and their individual volatile constituents: a review." *Phytotherapy Research*, 21(4): 308–323.
- Ostad, S.N. et al. (2001). "Pharmacological studies of *Foeniculum vulgare* essential oil and its major component, trans-anethole." *Darú Journal of Pharmaceutical Sciences*, 9(4): 73–77.
- Suhail, M.M. et al. (2011). "Chemical composition and therapeutic properties of *Boswellia carterii* essential oil." *BMC Complementary and Alternative Medicine*, 11(1):129.
- Ammon, H.P.T. (2010). "Modulation of the immune system by Boswellia serrata extracts and boswellic acids." *Phytomedicine*, 17(11): 862–867.
- Hammer, K.A. et al. (1999). "Antimicrobial activity of essential oils and other plant extracts." *Journal of Applied Microbiology*, 86(6): 985–990.
- Chrubasik, S. et al. (2005). "Zingiberis rhizoma: A comprehensive review on the ginger plant and its medicinal uses." *Phytomedicine*, 12(9): 684–701.
- Lakshmi, B. et al. (2011). "Pharmacological activities of Zingiber officinale (Ginger) and its active constituents." *Natural Product Communications*, 6(10): 1567–1577.
- Dorman, H.J.D., & Deans, S.G. (2000). "Antimicrobial agents from plants: antibacterial activity of plant volatile oils." *Journal of Applied Microbiology*, 88(2): 308–316.
- Koulivand, P.H., Khaleghi Ghadiri, M., & Gorji, A. (2013). "Lavender and the nervous system." *Evidence-*

Based Complementary and Alternative Medicine, 2013: 681304.

- Kamatou, G.P.P., Vermaak, I., & Viljoen, A.M. (2013). "Lemon (*Citrus limon*) essential oil: A review." *Phytochemistry Reviews*, 12: 801–820.
- Fisher, K., & Phillips, C. (2006). "Potential antimicrobial uses of citrus oils." *Food Control*, 17(10): 984–989.
- Hongratanaworakit, T. (2009). "Relaxing effect of marjoram oil inhalation on physiological parameters." *Journal of Medical Association of Thailand*, 92(2): 287–292.
- Buchbauer, G. et al. (1993). "Fragrance compounds and essential oils with sedative effects upon inhalation." *Journal of Pharmaceutical Sciences*, 82(6): 660–664.
- Cavanagh, H.M.A., & Wilkinson, J.M. (2002). "Biological activities of Neroli essential oil." *Phytotherapy Research*, 16(4): 301–308.
- Kamatou, G.P.P., Vermaak, I., & Viljoen, A.M. (2013). "Orange (*Citrus sinensis*) essential oil: Chemical composition and therapeutic properties." *Phytochemistry Reviews*, 12: 801–820.
- Fisher, K., & Phillips, C. (2006). "Potential antimicrobial uses of citrus oils." *Food Control*, 17(10): 984–989.
- Lis-Balchin, M. (2006). *Aromatherapy Science: A Guide for Healthcare Professionals*. Pharmaceutical Press.
- Dharmananda, S. (2003). "Palmarosa (*Cymbopogon martinii*): Botanical and therapeutic profile." *Institute for Traditional Medicine Review*.
- McKay, D.L., & Blumberg, J.B. (2006). "A review of the bioactivity and potential health benefits of peppermint tea (*Mentha piperita* L.)." *Phytotherapy Research*, 20(8): 619–633.
- Hwang, E., & Shin, S. (2018). "Menthol-rich peppermint essential oil: pharmacological properties and uses." *Journal of Ethnopharmacology*, 210: 242–251.

- Lis-Balchin, M. (2006). *Aromatherapy Science: A Guide for Healthcare Professionals*. Pharmaceutical Press.
- Jirovetz, L. et al. (2006). "Chemical composition and antimicrobial activity of Patchouli oil (*Pogostemon cablin*)." *Journal of Essential Oil Research*, 18(5): 556–560.
- Dorman, H.J.D., & Deans, S.G. (2000). "Antimicrobial agents from plants: antibacterial activity of plant volatile oils." *Journal of Applied Microbiology*, 88(2): 308–316.
- Buchbauer, G. et al. (1993). "Fragrance compounds and essential oils with sedative effects upon inhalation." *Journal of Pharmaceutical Sciences*, 82(6): 660–664.
- Buchbauer, G. et al. (1993). "Fragrance compounds and essential oils with sedative effects upon inhalation." *Journal of Pharmaceutical Sciences*, 82(6): 660–664.
- Cavanagh, H.M.A., & Wilkinson, J.M. (2002). "Biological activities of Rose essential oil." *Phytotherapy Research*, 16(4): 301–308.

About the Authors:

Dr. Nikhil Govind, B.Sc. (Biology), BNYS

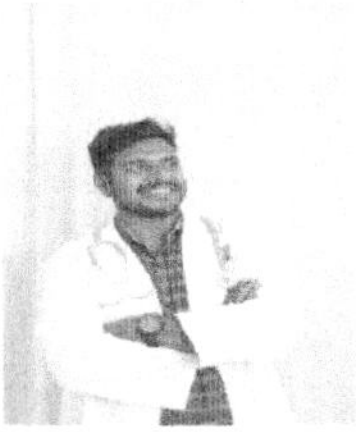

Dr. Nikhil Govind is a dedicated clinician, educator, and researcher in the field of **Naturopathy and holistic healing**. With several years of experience in naturopathy, therapeutic rehabilitation, and natural medicine, he has trained and guided many students in understanding the principles of natural healing and the therapeutic use of herbs and essential oils.

Having a strong academic background in **Biology and Naturopathy**, Dr. Nikhil Govind combines scientific knowledge with traditional healing wisdom. His work focuses on integrating natural therapies with modern health concepts, emphasizing **holistic wellness, preventive healthcare, and patient-centered healing**.

Dr. Nikhil Govind has actively contributed to **clinical training, academic teaching, and practical education** in the field of naturopathy and natural therapies. He is particularly interested in areas such as **aromatherapy, hydrotherapy, herbal medicine, and lifestyle-based healing approaches**. Through his teaching, workshops, and academic activities, he strives to make natural therapies more accessible and understandable for students and practitioners.

He is also the author of the book **"The Therapeutic Touch,"** which focuses on manipulative therapies and the science of manual healing techniques. That work reflects his dedication to teaching the art and precision of therapeutic touch. The present book, **"Herbal Essence,"** is his **second publication**, expanding his contribution to the field by exploring the healing power of aromatherapy and plant-based essential oils.

Known for his clear teaching style and commitment to holistic health, Dr. Nikhil Govind continues to inspire learners to appreciate the healing power of nature and apply it responsibly in clinical practice.

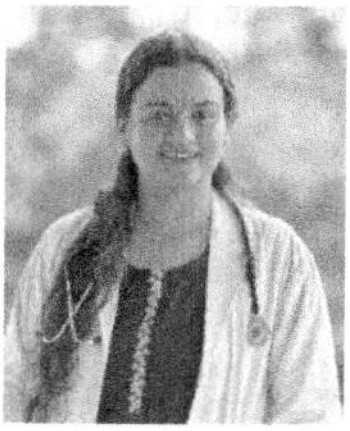

Dr Sandhya D, BNYS

Dr. Sandhya is a committed academic and skilled clinician in the field of manipulative therapy. With a strong foundation in anatomy and physiotherapy,
she blends scientific precision with therapeutic insight. Her teaching experience
and clinical practice reflect a deep dedication to empowering students and

advancing manual healing techniques. This book embodies her passion for structured learning, ethical care, and the transformative power of touch.

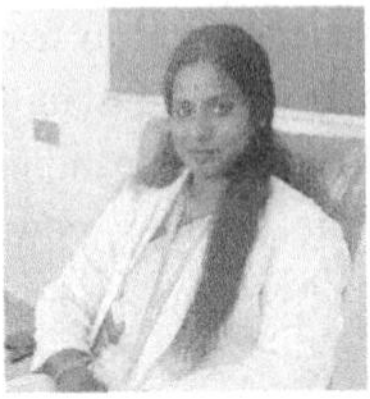

Harshitha M, Bsc(biotechnology),Msc(medical biochemistry)

Harshitha M holds a Bachelor's degree in Biotechnology and a Master's in Medical Biochemistry. With a strong foundation in life sciences and human physiology, she brings analytical depth and academic clarity to her work. Her
passion for integrative health and scientific education is reflected in her contributions to therapeutic and wellness literature.

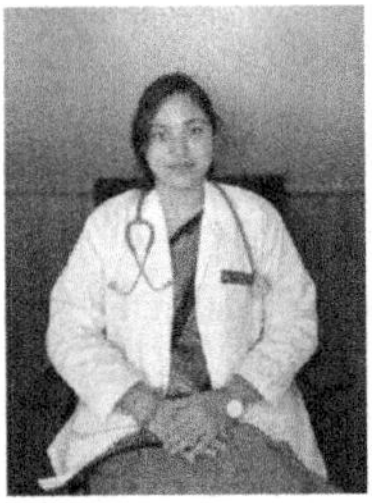

Dr. SOWJANYA, BNYS, MSc DFSM,

Dr. Sowjanya is a renowned clinician and researcher in naturopathy and yoga with over a decade of experience. With expertise in nutrition, chiropractic, yoga, and research, blends traditional holistic healing with modern diagnostics in clinical practice and education. Dr. Sowjanya has trained numerous students in naturopathic clinical practices and diagnostic techniques, shaping evidence-based holistic healthcare professionals. Contributions to curriculum development, academic programs, and professional education have been significant.
Through workshops, lectures, and publications, inspires students and practitioners to adopt a holistic approach to health and wellness, focusing on preventive healthcare, research, and natural healing systems.

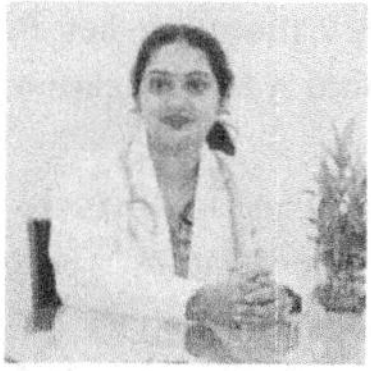

Dr. Ansa Anet Philip, BNYS

Dr. Ansa Anet Philip is a practitioner of Naturopathy and holistic health care with a strong interest in natural healing and wellness. She is dedicated to promoting health through aromatherapy, lifestyle medicine, and nature-based therapies.

With experience in clinical practice and patient care, Dr. Ansa Anet Philip focuses on encouraging holistic approaches for maintaining physical and mental well-being. As the co-author of "Herbal Essence," she contributes her knowledge and interest in aromatherapy and the therapeutic use of essential oils.

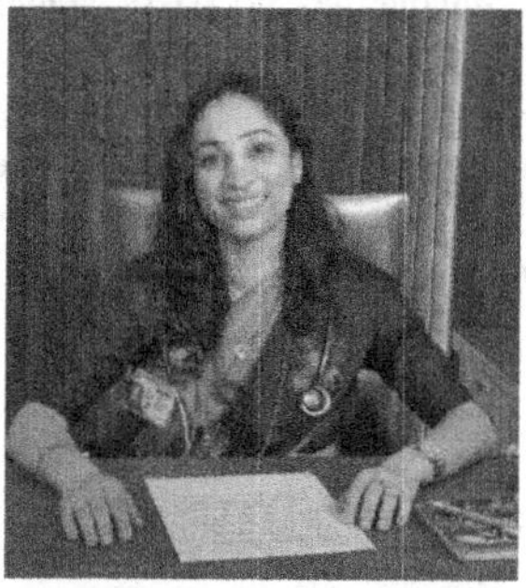

Dr Vinutha Rao BNYS,Msc,(Phd)

Dr. Vinutha Rao, BNYS, MSc (Clinical Nutrition & Dietetics) is the **Principal of MVM College of Naturopathy & Yogic Sciences, Bangalore**, and an **Hon'ble Governor-nominated Senate Member of Rajiv Gandhi University of Health Sciences (RGUHS)**. She holds the distinction of being the **first female BNYS member nominated to the Senate**.

She completed her **BNYS from Alva's College of Naturopathy & Yogic Sciences** and obtained her **Master's degree in Clinical Nutrition and**

Dietetics from KSOU, Mysore. She is currently **pursuing her PhD in Integrated Nutrition** and also an **MBA in Hospital Administration**.

Dr. Vinutha Rao began her clinical practice in **2009** and has **over 16 years of experience** in clinical practice, research, and academics. During her professional career, she has served in several reputed institutions including **Jindal Nature Cure Institute, Bangalore**, **Health Care Global Enterprises (HCG)**, **Government Yoga and Naturopathy Centre at Jaya Chamarajendra Hospital, Arsikere**, and **Nisarga Nature Cure Hospital, Sirsi**.

She is an **invited speaker at national and international conferences**, conducts **Yoga and Naturopathy workshops for organizations**, and has participated in various public health awareness programs. She has also presented several **radio programs** and published articles in newspapers and magazines such as **Health Herald** and **Heritage Amruth**.

Dr. Vinutha Rao has received several recognitions including the **WOW Award (2016)**, **Best Doctor Award by Sri Jindal (2018)**, and the **Corona Warrior Award from Rotary Club** for her dedicated service. She has also been **felicitated for her contributions during the COVID-19 pandemic**.

She currently serves as the **Secretary of the Indian Naturopathy and Yoga Graduates Medical Association (INYGMA), Karnataka Chapter**, and the **President of the Alva's Alumni Association**, actively contributing to the advancement of Naturopathy and Yogic Sciences.

About the Editor

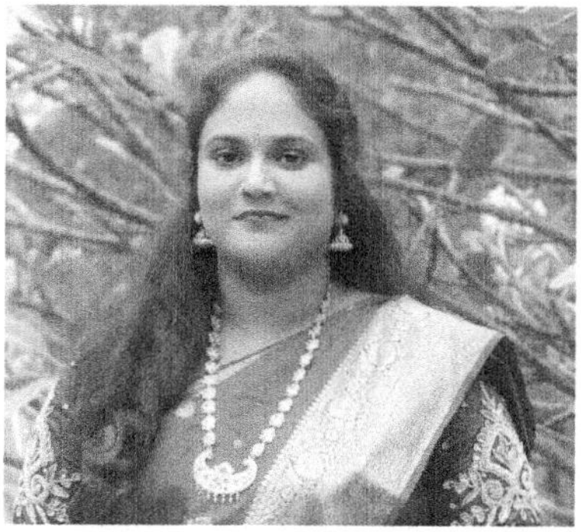

Mrs. K. R. Rohini Das, BE, M.Tech, (PhD) is an academician and researcher with a strong background in **engineering, research, and academic development**. With extensive experience in teaching and scholarly work, she has been actively involved in guiding students and contributing to academic publications.

Her expertise in **research methodology, academic writing, and technical editing** has enabled her to support and refine scholarly works across various disciplines. Known for her attention to detail and commitment to academic excellence, she plays a significant role in ensuring clarity, accuracy, and quality in academic publications.

As the **editor of the book "Herbal Essence,"** Ms. Rohini Das has contributed to shaping the manuscript with clarity and precision, helping present the concepts of aromatherapy and natural healing in a structured and reader-friendly manner.